BREASTFEEDING
AND NATURAL CHILD SPACING

After her graduation as a dental hygienist from the University of California Medical Center in San Francisco, Sheila Kippley married and began raising a family. She became interested in breastfeeding following the birth of her first child. A few years later, when her husband's work had taken her to Canada, she started a La Leche League group whose members often questioned her about breastfeeding and its relationship to child spacing. As a result, she began collecting material to help mothers and eventually wrote *Breastfeeding and Natural Child Spacing*. In the fall of 1971 she and her husband founded the Couple to Couple League which helps couples to learn the art of natural family planning. Mrs. Kippley is the mother of five children.

Cover photo: Sheila Kippley with daughter Karen, 1972.

Breastfeeding and Natural Child Spacing

How "Ecological" Breastfeeding Spaces Babies

Sheila K. Kippley

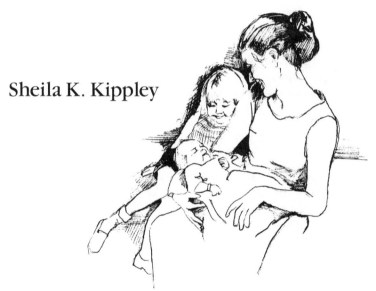

Drawings by Gigi Nealon

Second Revised Edition

The Couple to Couple League International, Inc.
Cincinnati

Publisher
The Couple to Couple League International, Inc.
Location
3621 Glenmore Avenue
Cincinnati, Ohio
Mailing address
P.O. Box 111184
Cincinnati, OH 45211
U.S.A.

Preliminary edition: K Publishers, 1969
First edition: Harper and Row Publishers, Inc., New York, 1974
Paperback edition: Penquin Books Inc., 1975

Cataloging data

Kippley, Sheila K.
Breastfeeding and Natural Child Spacing: How "Ecological" Breastfeeding Spaces Babies

1. Breastfeeding   2. Parenting
3. Natural family planning   4. Family planning
5. Birth control

ISBN 0-9601036-8-6 (previously ISBN 0-1400-3992-9)

Acknowledgements

This book could not have been written in its present form without the help of others. Thus I want to thank all of the publishers who graciously gave me permission to quote from their publications. The many mothers who told me their experiences either personally or by mail made an invaluable contribution to the writing of this book. To each of them I express my deep thanks. Many readers will recognize that I have been influenced by La Leche League. I freely and gratefully acknowledge my great debt to that organization, and I certainly thank those League members and officials who have helped me in various ways.

There are several individuals who have been of special help in preparing the revised edition. Linda Langlitz did me a great favor by reviewing the entire revised manuscript and offering helpful suggestions. And I certainly want to thank the women at the CCL office — Betty Schwartz, Dorthea Farrell, Virginia Niehaus, and Rosemay Olding for their help in the sometimes tedious tasks of word processing and proofreading. Lastly, my husband, John, first suggested that I breastfeed our babies, and his aid in preparing both the original manuscript and this revised edition was indeed significant.

Contents

Some Important Addresses

The following organizations are frequently referred to in the text:

For breastfeeding information

La Leche League International (LLLI)
P. O. Box 1209
Franklin Park, IL 60131-8209
Counseling telephone number at any time: (312) 455-7730

For childbirth information

NAPSAC*
Rt 1, Box 646
Marble Hill, MO 63764
(314) 238-2010

*National Association of Parents and Professionals for Safe Alternatives in Childbirth

For natural family planning information

The Couple to Couple League
P. O. Box 111184
Cincinnati, OH 45211-1184
(513) 661-7612

For materials recommended in this book, please see the mini-catalog at the back of the book.

Introduction

This manual is a book of its times. A hundred years ago it would have been superfluous because breastfeeding was the general practice, and it would have been impossible because of the lack of research at that time. Today, however, I think it fills a need.

The book grew out of a great many conversations I had with other mothers who shared with me a common interest in providing our babies with the benefits of breastfeeding and in securing the additional side effect of child spacing. All of us ran up against what seemed to be a nearly universal skepticism about both of these common interests—at least at the level of homemaker hearsay. On the other hand, at the level of medical research, our common interests were bolstered. When I frequently found myself playing the role of transmitter of scientific information about breastfeeding and child spacing, I decided that there was a general knowledge gap on the part of many mothers and doctors that might be narrowed by a book of this type.

More importantly, the methods advocated in this manual provided a double service to friends of mine who had previously been unsuccessful in their earlier attempts at breastfeeding. First of all, they become successful nursing mothers and, as a result, came to a greater enjoyment of their babies. Secondly, they experienced a form of child spacing for which they were not only appreciative but which some of them had believed could not be achieved through nursing.

The particular information that I as well as others needed clarification about was the possibility of becoming pregnant while nursing. I came to the realization that some mothers who sincerely wanted to continue to breastfeed their babies were weaning very early for fear of pregnancy following soon after childbirth. Some of these fears were real because of cultural interference with natural breastfeeding; almost all were the result of inadequate information. I found that a review of the medical research in this area, plus the adoption of the breastfeeding and child-care program described in this manual, gave some mothers of my acquaintance confidence, peace of mind, and the enjoyment of continued nursing.

I want to stress at the outset that breastfeeding is far more than a merely biological function. It is frequently an emotional experience for both mother and baby; it is truly interpersonal. The breastfeeding mother is not just fulfilling a mammary function; she is also contributing to the personal fulfillment of herself as a mother and to the emotional security and development of her baby. This is part of what is meant by "the ecology of natural mothering," a theme that runs throughout this book.

This is not a book on birth control as such, although I fully realize that some may be interested in what is said here primarily from the point of view of finding an efficient means of child spacing that meets the moral criteria of everyone. It is not within the scope of this book to delve deeply into a values discussion; rather, the purpose here is to show that, for whatever reason breastfeeding is used, it can be an effective means of spacing children. I will say, however, that the more the mother thinks in terms of doing what is most in accord with nature and what is best for her baby, the more easily she will be able to carry out the program outlined here. Furthermore, it is somewhat doubtful whether the mother who would look at breastfeeding only as a means of birth control would be able to sustain the criticism she might get from her well-meaning friends and advisers. And one doesn't become a member of the smart set by extended breastfeeding although some extremely smart women are doing it. Breastfeeding entails a loving personal relationship between mother and baby, and I wonder if the mother who looked upon her suckling baby primarily as a birth-control device would be able to maintain that nursing relationship of love for very long. Psychological studies have indicated that a baby can sense his mother's attitude toward him from the way in which she nurses him,* and no one would want to see such a naturally loving relationship distorted. For the mother who may start out with a poor attitude toward her child, however, I think that with a little bit of self-giving there is a much greater chance of her growing to accept, love, and appreciate her baby through breastfeeding than through the use of such artifacts as bottles, formulas, messy baby foods, and pacifiers.

---

*Readers will notice that I refer to the baby as masculine. Many sentences and paragraphs talk about both the mother and baby, and it is much easier to keep the pronouns straight by referring to the baby as he, him, and his.

I hope that no one will take offense at my efforts to paraphrase the Man from Nazareth. Speaking of the relationship of secular values and the kingdom of God, He said, "Seek first the kingdom of God and all these other things will be given unto you." What I have been trying to say is that, by seeking first to do what is in accord with God's natural plan, other benefits will follow.

Readers of the previous edition will note the following differences. First of all, five chapters have been added. Secondly, all the chapters have undergone at least some small changes, and some chapters have been changed significantly. Third, an appendix dealing with an extensive review of the pre-1974 research has been eliminated. It is refreshing to note that what was a rather controversial position in the late sixties and early seventies has now become widely accepted among scientific experts as well as among mothers who experience it—namely, that what we call ecological breastfeeding normally provides an extended duration of postpartum infertility.

Lastly, more attention is given to the transition from breastfeeding infertility to the process of systematic natural family planning. To put it another way, in this edition I've provided more detail on how to detect the eventual return of your fertility while breastfeeding.

In summary, this book has been written so that mothers will come to enjoy the same satisfying relationship with their babies that I have experienced. I hope that they will also, if that is what they want, come to enjoy the derivative effect of natural child spacing. At the least, they and whoever else is interested will learn about some of the research that has been done concerning breastfeeding and natural infertility, what is meant by natural mothering, its many advantages for the individual baby and mother, and its normal effect of child spacing.

1

Your Baby's Sucking Needs

THE BREAST FOR NOURISHMENT

One of a baby's strongest needs is the need to suck—and rightly so, for it's his primary means of obtaining nourishment in the early weeks and months after birth. The nursing of an infant stimulates the production of milk in his mother and is the natural means of transmitting milk from mother to baby.

Lactation, or the production of milk in the mother's body, is influenced proportionately by the amount of stimulation the breast receives. This stimulation is most frequently caused by the nursing of the infant. (Another source of stimulation that is not as strong as that caused by the infant is expression of milk by hand or pump.) The more stimulation the breast receives, the more milk it will supply or produce. The exact opposite is likewise true. When a baby weans himself gradually from the breast or is weaned by his mother who introduces foods or formula so that her baby requires less from the breast, then her supply of milk is lessened accordingly. Lactation is a delicate process, for the supply of milk almost always meets the demands, whether that demand is great or small.

The following story illustrates how a mother's milk supply is influenced largely by her baby's demand at the breast. A friend introduced solids early at the advice of her doctor. Unlike her previous doctor, this new doctor insisted on solids at six weeks even though he strongly approved of breastfeeding. As soon as she followed his instructions, her milk supply decreased, she became depressed, and menstruation returned. Several months later a let-

1

ter came, telling me that her supply had increased.

Of course, I'm still nursing Jeff. He only has solids once a day. Frank and I both felt we should cut down on solids, and we had a good chance to do so over the Easter holidays when we traveled to Salt Lake. He had very little extra, and I feel this brought back or brought on more milk. Makes me happier.

It is amazing at first to learn how effective the demand for milk can be in producing the supply. There are mothers who want to bring back their milk several months after childbirth because their babies have reacted unfavorably to formulas. With proper instruction and loads of encouragement, these mothers have brought back their supply and have been able to breastfeed their babies.

The same process can likewise assist the mother who, worried at first about an insufficient milk supply and deciding her baby perhaps needed a supplement via a bottle, would like to eliminate that supplementary bottle. By doubling or tripling the number of nursings at the breast for one or two days, the mother will usually have plenty of milk, and there will be no further need to use the bottle.

Another example is the mother who has a premature or sick baby. She may express her milk regularly to maintain a supply until her baby comes home. Over a period of six weeks one mother expressed her milk into a sterile jar which she took daily to the hospital to nourish her premature, incubator baby. Her supply increased from one and one-half ounces to over twenty ounces per day during this period. She met up with much resistance at first, and everyone thought it wasn't possible. At a later date the pediatrician told her to wean the baby to a bottle by six months of age, his reason being that the nursing wouldn't do her or the baby any good. Being well read on the subject of breastfeeding, she ignored this advice and both she and the baby prospered.

A few mothers have produced milk for the baby they planned to adopt. I have corresponded with one mother who actually was producing milk prior to adoption. In another case the mother had not recently given birth; she was without any supply of milk and she was without the normal hormonal and physiological changes of late pregnancy that provide an adequate and easy milk supply after childbirth. She was, so to speak, bone dry, yet she persevered and developed a milk supply for her adopted baby.

Needless to say, such a process isn't recommended to just anybody, for it takes a considerable amount of constant effort and a very strong desire to nurse one's baby. In addition, it takes a baby who is agreeable to the idea, for by the time an adoptive mother

2

receives her baby, the infant may have been bottle-fed for several weeks. It takes more work to get milk from the breast than from the bottle, and some babies are not particularly disposed toward making the transition.

Nature also provides an ample supply of milk to those mothers who have twins. One doctor insisted that his patient nurse her twin babies because he felt it would be easier for her. I have a friend who had two sets of twins and found this to be true. It is the only way a mother can feed two babies at the same time!

In addition, a few mothers with one breast have been encouraged by their doctors to nurse in order to reduce the chance of developing cancer in the remaining breast. The American Cancer Society and the National Cancer Institute of the USPH Service report that cancer of the breast is more apt to develop in those breasts that do not give milk, and scientific studies confirm the fact that long-term nursing lowers the breast-cancer risk.

These examples are given to show you not only how lactation can be encouraged under unusual or different circumstances but above all to impress upon you, as a mother, that you certainly can nurse your baby under normal conditions. The important thing to remember is that breastfeeding can be a very easy and natural affair. God gave you your baby and He also provided you with the best food for your baby, food that you alone can give him. To help you feed your baby, He gave your infant a strong urge to suck. It's that simple. Let the baby nurse often at the breast, and you will have plenty of milk for nourishment.

THE BREAST AS A PACIFIER

This brings us to another important point. Babies have an obvious need to suck. They will suck on anything they come in contact with—breast, fingers, clothing, or objects. This is a normal, healthy habit that should be encouraged (the baby or older child will outgrow it easily later if his desire to suck isn't frustrated early in life); it's a need that is particularly well satisfied at his mother's breast.

The breast is nature's pacifier for the baby. This is hard for many mothers to appreciate in our culture where bottle-feeding shares equal status with breastfeeding and where the bottle is preferred when a feeding takes place outside the home. We tend to ignore the fact that these artificial aids—bottles and pacifiers—are merely substitutes for mother. The infant's need to be pacified at the breast is nature's way of bringing mother and baby together at other than feeding times. The breast produces the same effect as a bottle or a soother—that is, it calms the infant, which is often the way the baby likes to feel before going to sleep. The breastfed baby wants the breast for this "pacifying" need of his just as a bottle-fed baby prefers his bottle or soother. This is why the nursing mother cannot really say how many times she has fed her baby during the day. Does she count the times she has pacified her baby into a deep sleep—even though her baby might have acquired little milk in the process? The breast also offers security and comfort. It brings love and reassurance any time during the day or night.

Suckling is also apparently a very satisfying experience in itself. Dr. James Hymes, author of the *The Child Under Six*[1], says that suckling provides babies with many pleasant sensations, and in *The First Nine Months*[2], Geraldine Lux Flanagan points out that some babies are born with a callus on their thumbs as a result of their sucking activity in the womb. Surely this is an indication that sucking was a satisfying experience for these babies even before birth.

Perhaps this is a good place to begin to explain what is meant by the subtitle of this book, "How Ecological Breastfeeding Spaces Babies." Strictly speaking, ecology is concerned with the relationship between living things and their environment. Frequently it is a rather delicate relationship, and every year we read about how this or that animal or fish or tree may be affected by such and such a change in the environment. The language of ecology is applied

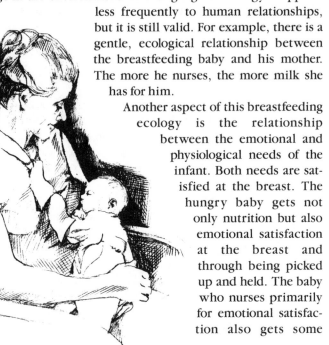

less frequently to human relationships, but it is still valid. For example, there is a gentle, ecological relationship between the breastfeeding baby and his mother. The more he nurses, the more milk she has for him.

Another aspect of this breastfeeding ecology is the relationship between the emotional and physiological needs of the infant. Both needs are satisfied at the breast. The hungry baby gets not only nutrition but also emotional satisfaction at the breast and through being picked up and held. The baby who nurses primarily for emotional satisfaction also gets some nourishment and simultaneously helps reinforce his mother's milk supply. The mother can continue to satisfy the emotional need at the breast even when her baby has a nutritional need for other foods in addition to breast milk. This helps to explain why some cultures that are sensitive to the child's needs think nothing of continuing partial breastfeeding for three or more years.

Breastfeeding plays an important role in the emotional development of the mother, too. The nursing relationship can give her a feeling of self-importance and self-worth as a mother from the satisfaction gained in meeting her baby's needs herself. The rewards in giving, especially to one's small children, are emotional ones that cannot be measured.

Last but not least, the frequent stimulation of the breast by the baby plays an extremely important role in maintaining natural infertility after childbirth. Frequency of suckling appears to be the most important factor in maintaining breastfeeding infertility. Such frequency is brought about by satisfying your baby's needs—both nutritional and emotional—at your breast. This and other aspects of the breastfeeding ecology will be spelled out in later chapters. Suffice it to say for now that Mother Nature has provided a mutually beneficial relationship in breastfeeding and provides many opportunities for its proper development.

SUCKING STIMULUS AND OVULATION

When a young girl reaches puberty, she normally begins to experience the menstrual cycle. If she has prepared for this as a natural development, she accepts it as part of becoming an adult woman and may give it little further thought. On the other hand, she may have wanted a better understanding of her bodily functions and sought out the whole story behind her monthly cycle. If you are such a woman, the following facts will scarcely be new; but certain facts take on new relevance when seen in relation to childbearing and child spacing.

A baby girl at birth has two ovaries which contain all the eggs (or ova) that she will ever have. At puberty her ovaries become active, and during each fertility-menstrual cycle an egg develops and approaches the surface of the ovary. When its individual container called a follicle ruptures, the egg or ovum is released from the ovary and is now free to travel from the ovary down the Fallopian tubes toward the womb or uterus. The release of an ovum is necessary before fertilization or conception can take place and is called ovulation.

While your body is preparing for ovulation, the lining of your uterus is thickening to receive the newly conceived human life should conception occur. If the ovum is not fertilized, the lining of the uterus is sloughed off and bleeding occurs. This bleeding is known as menstruation or menses, and it's often referred to as a "menstrual period."

If pregnancy occurs, however, a change occurs in the body chemistry. One effect of this is that the lining of the womb is not sloughed off but remains built up, thereby eliminating menstrual bleeding during pregnancy. This is termed pregnancy amenorrhea. **Amenorrhea** simply means "not having periods." Another effect of this change in the body chemistry during pregnancy is that the ovaries remain at rest; no ovulation and no additional pregnancy can occur until after childbirth. The only exception would be multiple conceptions; but it is known that when double or triple ovulations occur in a cycle, they all occur within the same twenty-four hour period.

Our interest in this whole process is the continuation of this infertile condition following childbirth. If the mother nurses her baby properly, she will normally retain this infertile condition by experiencing a lengthy absence from menstrual periods following birth. This is known as lactation amenorrhea. The medical researchers have been unable to describe with certainty the body chemistry involved, but there is widespread agreement that the frequent nursing by the infant at the breast is the most important factor in providing this natural infertility.

There are two practical conclusions for the nursing mother who would like the side benefit of breastfeeding infertility. First of all, she should positively cooperate with her baby's natural desires to nurse whether it be for nutritional or emotional needs. Secondly, she should avoid those practices that prematurely lessen her baby's feeding at the breast. This would include almost the entire range of cultural baby-care practices in the United States: early solids and liquids other than mother's milk, rigid nursing schedules, pacifiers, the race to get baby sleeping through the night, baby-sitters, and so on.

The guidelines that are given in this book go hand in hand with what I call "natural mothering." By natural mothering I mean that care of an infant in which his needs are met primarily by his mother and not by artifacts or baby-sitters. It is natural baby care as well, for the mother follows her baby's natural development or pattern. Natural mothering, then, is not ruled by clocks or schedules; instead, the baby is the mother's guide.

It is one thing to state the guidelines for natural spacing; it is something else to put a natural mothering program into practice in the face of some current customs of child care. Unfortunately, many of the current practices today restrict or eliminate the mothering that nature intended and seriously interfere with the natural infertility of breastfeeding. Because these factors take the baby away from his mother, some of the following chapters will look at these cultural practices in more detail to see how they hinder nature's plan for spacing babies.

References

1. James Hymes, *The Child Under Six* (Englewood Cliffs: Prentice-Hall, 1963).
2. Geraldine Lux Flanagan, *The First Nine Months* (New York: Pocket Books, 1962).

2

Does Complete Mean Total?

In the last chapter the infertility of pregnancy was compared with the infertility of breastfeeding, and the absence of ovulation and menstruation was noted in both. It's obvious that the baby developing in his mother's womb derives 100 percent of his nourishment from his mother. The point that cannot be overstressed with regard to breastfeeding and ovulation is that the baby who gives his mother the natural infertility of breastfeeding will also be getting 100 percent of his nourishment from his mother's breast, at least during the first six months. Less than 100 percent is weaning,* and nowhere do I want to give the impression that breastfeeding plus supplements in the early months provides the same degree of infertility that complete or total breastfeeding does.

---

* Weaning refers to the process of introducing a breastfed baby to other foods or liquids. This process can last two days, two weeks, twelve months, or three years. It begins as soon as the mother offers her baby something else for nourishment besides breast milk; it ends the day that her baby no longer takes any milk from the breast. From this definition, it can be said that many mothers wean their babies from the day they leave the hospital, even though they actually nurse for six or ten months. In addition, the baby also undergoes an emotional weaning off the breast, gradually receiving this emotional nourishment in other ways from his mother and from other sources and contacts.

In a society conditioned to look to physicians for help in every phase of life, and especially in the areas of infant nutrition, it is difficult to be understood when speaking about complete breast-feeding. Complete breastfeeding doesn't require any formulas, any juice, any baby foods, or any special concoctions. (I am not considering the case of the sick baby who may need special treatment. I am speaking only about the normal healthy baby.) However, the fact is that in the fifties and sixties most doctors prescribed formulas and set up definite schedules for the introduction of juices, liquids, cereals, and solids—and some still do. Thus mothers came to believe that this was medically, nutritionally, and psychologically the "best" way, and breastfeeding was either looked down upon as fit for only the lower social groups or as a nice but very short-run supplement to the "real" nourishment put out by the food and drug companies.

Complete or total breastfeeding means, again, that the baby derives all his food from his mother's breasts. It means that the only nipples that need to be in the house are part of his mother's natural equipment. It should go without saying that there does not have to be a baby bottle in the house.

Now I have nothing against the mother who bottle-feeds or who partially breastfeeds. My only complaint comes when the mother who partially breastfeeds tells her friends that she is nursing and that, of course, her menstrual periods have started or that she became pregnant. I want to agree with the "of course," but I also want to make it clear that her partial breastfeeding is what I call weaning, not total or complete breastfeeding.

If I seem somewhat repetitious on this point, it's because I am convinced that misunderstanding is so widespread that a single statement is not sufficient. Perhaps the following examples will illustrate why I think the idea needs clarification.

In 1967 a mother wrote to *Our Sunday Visitor* saying that if breastfeeding "is done properly it will suspend ovulation and menstruation for seven to fifteen months." She encouraged other mothers to give it a try, as "it is still God's plan for spacing babies." Some letters were printed several weeks later showing the various responses to her letter. The following are excerpts from some of those letters.

"I know a mother who had nine children in eleven years; she breastfed each until a new pregnancy forced her to stop. . ."

"I also have a friend who is a nurse and breastfeeds every baby and in six years has had four babies and two miscarriages. . ."

"I think probably a mother who nurses during the first three months would suppress ovulation but not for seven to fifteen months . . . and then only if it is complete nursing with no supplement foods, and most doctors would want you to start other foods at least by three months."

A close friend sent me the newspaper clippings of these letters with a note attached: "I think that these ladies who object to nursing as a natural baby spacer probably don't know enough about it. I mean about no solids or supplements."

One time after I had just finished explaining total breastfeeding to a mother she said, "Well, that can't be true. I nursed and still had my periods." After I asked her a few more questions, she said, "Oh, yes. I gave a bottle to my babies."

Another mother gave a similar response after being told about the spacing benefit of breastfeeding. "Well, I nursed my babies for ten months and always had periods." She was asked if she gave the baby anything else. "Oh, yes," she said, "you don't expect a baby to get along on just breast milk, do you?"

And a mother who expressed an interest in natural child spacing referred to herself, after some discussion, as "only nursing;" yet earlier in the conversation she had mentioned giving her baby several bottles of juice during the day to keep the baby on a four-hour schedule.

Mothers who become interested in natural child spacing eventually find themselves talking about this aspect of breastfeeding with their friends and relatives. Most of their acquaintances will admit that they do not remember when they introduced solids or the bottle or when they nursed their babies, nor do they remember when their periods returned. Some mothers, however, do insist that they became pregnant while nursing, but usually later conversations bring out the fact that they were weaning at the time of conception. One mother insisted on several different occasions that she became pregnant while only nursing her baby, but later talked about how she gave solids to her babies at three months. As her relative told her, "There you go. There's your answer. You weren't completely nursing." Another mother insisted likewise, but it was later learned that she gave supplementary feedings a few weeks after the birth of her babies. A third mother who was sure that she became pregnant while completely nursing later said that she was giving her baby "only juice at the time." These actual remarks convince me that many people do not understand what is meant by complete or total breastfeeding.

I consider myself more fortunate than many. With our first child the obstetrician discouraged me with regard to breastfeeding, and especially with regard to its natural effect of spacing babies. He was very firm and negative on this point, and I accepted his views.

However, with our second child I had a different obstetrician who listened to my desire to nurse the baby and to my questions about child spacing through breastfeeding. He affirmed the spacing effect, but only if I nursed totally. He told me to use nothing but breast milk to nourish the baby. I remember asking him, "What about water?" And he answered, "Not even water." I was told to nurse my baby in this manner for as long as I desired—and I found this most welcome advice.

The truth of the matter is that when a mother provides 1) all of her baby's nourishment at her breast and 2) the greater part of his other sucking needs at her breast, she will almost invariably experience the side effect of natural infertility. You can have child spacing (using other means) without breastfeeding, but you cannot normally have breastfeeding in the sense described above without the side effect of child spacing. To put it another way, if a woman should sincerely want to become pregnant within six months following childbirth, she should not follow the breastfeeding plan described in this chapter.

I want to call special attention to the second part of the statement above in boldface type, "the greater part of his other sucking needs." Some mothers have been very disappointed to experience menstruation or conception while totally breastfeeding. Too often, however, these mothers are restricting the nursing by not following the other aspects of natural mothering. In other words, the total breastfeeding rule is no guarantee that menstruation or ovulation will not occur. A mother who follows the total breastfeeding *nutrition* rule may not be satisfying her child's other needs at the breast. May I give you a true example?

A breastfeeding mother phoned for information on natural family planning—information neither the hospital nor her doctor could give her. Knowing that she had nursed her babies, we discussed natural spacing. She wasn't initially interested in reading the material I had gathered on the subject, but I encouraged her to do so to see if she really was an exception—for she was convinced that she was the odd case. She had totally breastfed all her babies, yet experienced regular menstrual periods three and one- half to four weeks after childbirth with all six children. She never once experienced an absence of periods while nursing. In addition, she was nursing her sixth baby often, day and night. Upon returning the material, she wrote:

First an apology—someone had told me you were "far-out" and I accepted the opinion without investigation. Our problem in nursing probably lies in not letting Jane suck long enough. I usually have a fast flow. She is satisfied in about eight to ten minutes. I also have used both breasts to fill her up to save time. She sucks her finger, and this indicates a need for more sucking. I do nurse lying down as often as possible, but I've seldom let the baby fall asleep with me. I feel that my practice of nursing quickly also is at fault. Don't you? Let me try some of your suggestions and we'll see what happens."

The suggestions the mother was referring to were those in the material I had given her, as normally I do not suggest a change in nursing or mothering habits for those interested in natural family planning if menstruation has already occurred.

About six months later I happened to meet this mother and learned from her that she experienced lactation amenorrhea for the first time. Her baby was four months old when her periods stopped, and she went four months without menstrual bleeding. This particular case illustrates that there is much more to natural spacing than merely filling baby's tummy or satisfying hunger pangs by total breastfeeding.

In the past the total breastfeeding nutrition rule was the only guideline taught to mothers who were interested in nursing and in avoiding an immediate pregnancy. True, that rule is extremely important, but it's only one aspect of the overall natural spacing picture. Other guidelines are also important, and they deserve as much attention and emphasis.

3

New Light on Night Feedings

This topic does not appeal to many mothers, but it's an important one to consider if you are interested in natural child spacing. Night feedings are normal for a breastfed baby. Many infants need one night feeding—and oftentimes several—during the first or even the second year of life. These feedings are important for several reasons, the most obvious being that they form a part of the baby's nutrition. In line with that, it should be noted that the regularity of the nursing tends to produce a regular supply of milk. From the point of view of natural child spacing, night feedings are important because the frequent nursing which maintains an ample milk supply also is responsible for the natural spacing. A mother who anticipates that her breastfeeding will result in both a healthy baby and natural infertility will hardly go for ten or twelve hours without nursing during the day. She should likewise not set a goal of so many hours without nursing her baby during the night. The absence of a feeding for any length of time may initiate an early return of your menstrual periods and thereby shorten your breast-feeding infertility. If you want the natural child spacing effect of breastfeeding, then give your baby the night feedings he will naturally desire.

CONTEMPORARY SOCIAL ATTITUDES

Contemporary emphasis is placed on getting the baby to sleep all the way through the night and at the earliest possible date. The longer the baby sleeps at night, the better he is thought to be. Parents pride themselves on the speed with which they can get their new baby to sleep the entire night. They learn to fill up the baby before bedtime with the hope that this will satisfy him for the duration of the night. If the baby does wake, they hope that the fussing or crying will only be temporary, so that they will not have to get out of bed—for which no one can blame them. When those hopes fail and they have to get up, they might have to go to the bother of warming up a bottle; and by the time that chore is done—to the tune of the baby's crying—all they are hoping for is that the baby will feed himself back to sleep without further ado. But then there's the problem of the air that the baby took in from the bottle. Now he needs burping, and that means a second trip from the bed to baby. With this type of routine it's no wonder that bottle-feeding parents aim for that goal of "all through the night as early as possible."

Others hope to do the trick with the pacifier. As one mother put it rather bluntly, "Let's face it. We stick the pacifier back in their mouths, hoping they'll settle down and go back to sleep again." Another answer to the problem was recommended recently by a doctor to a friend of mine. He told the couple to put the baby in the bathroom, close the door, and let the baby cry it out.

The breastfeeding mother is likewise warned not to fall asleep while nursing or she will crush or smother her child. Thus, getting up to feed her baby becomes a tiresome chore, and she soon longs for a full night's rest. Under this regime for night feedings, the mother is most anxious to pry the baby off the breast as soon as she can and the nursing is very restricted.

The nursing mother is often instructed to wean the baby from night feedings at an early age. If the baby objects, she is often advised to ignore his cries. She may be told to offer him a bottle or to let her husband take care of the baby because all the baby wants is his mother anyway! One mother we know was advised by her doctor to give her two-month-old baby a drug so he would sleep through the night. At any rate, most babies sleep away from their mothers anyway, and they soon begin to learn to sleep through the night on their own. They never have the pleasure of receiving from their mother during the night hours that touch stimulation said to be so important.

The problem of night feeding, however, is partially eliminated by a change of attitudes, by simply looking to the best interests of the baby instead of to our own convenience. During my first three years of mothering, I happened to have frequent contact with a small group of women who placed a great deal of emphasis on the needs of their babies. Good mothering meant meeting baby's needs during the night as well as during the day. Therefore, it was common to hear a mother speak of night feedings when her child was twelve months old or even eighteen months old. When we moved, I soon learned that such a group was in the minority, that most people have entirely different views about raising children compared to those views I had acquired from my original exposure. In our new environment, it seemed that the question most frequently asked about our baby was: "Is she sleeping through the night now?" or "How often do you have to feed her during the night?" According to this viewpoint, night feedings are a problem to be conquered instead of simply part of the process of child care.

The answer to such questions is rather simple. Our children will never take a prize for all-night sleeping at an early age. My husband and I learned that this is one phase they outgrow when they are ready; and not only are there many advantages to both parent and baby in letting nature take its course in this area, but doing so eliminates all the worries and problems inherent in training a child to sleep through the night.

Our first two children awoke for night feedings every night until we decided that it might be time to stop this "habit." When they were both eighteen months old, we tried all the tricks and none worked. So we resorted to the "crying it out" scheme. That worked within two or three nights. We would never do it this way again if we had another chance, but at that time we were uninformed. We didn't really feel this was the best way, but we conformed to our society's norms and thus made our children also conform.

With our second child we discovered that sleeping with the baby was safe and we were becoming more open to the philosophy of the family bed. We grew even more with our third child; the family bed was a reality from the day of her birth, and we adopted the natural mothering/parenting lifestyle by following a more natural, child-centered approach. Accepting the family bed actually was the step that led us to accept changes in other areas of parenting. This book would have never been written if we had remained a two-child family.

While our intentions were right, sometimes it is more difficult to adjust to the family bed as the child turns one or two years old. My husband was slower to accept the family bed as our third child, then two years old, was still in our bed. He insisted one night that she stay in her bed during the night and placed her in a separate room and closed the door to soften the cries. The crying began, but it didn't last long. Our oldest daughter (then six years old) brought her to our bed since she couldn't stand it any longer, and the youngest stayed for many more nights.

Well past her third birthday she was still crawling into bed with us at some time during the wee hours for some nursing. There were a few times when we had our doubts, but at these times support came in one form or another.

Some of this support came in the form of writings which I will refer to later. Other support came through personal acquaintances and correspondence. I learned from a friend that her child, although weaned when ten months old, didn't sleep naturally through the night until she was four and a half years old. And in talking with mothers, I learned that many have a similar situation at night, regardless of whether they chose to bottle-feed or breast-feed. However, since babies are "supposed" to sleep through the night, many mothers do not admit it or like to talk about it. Likewise, I was fortunate to be able to correspond with other nursing mothers, and I found that there was always someone else who was night-nursing a baby older than ours. You can't imagine how much support this was!

We are pleased with the results. In our experience, taking care of the child's real needs at this early stage does not set a pattern for the development of an emotionally unstable child who is filled with all sorts of imagined needs later on. Quite the opposite. Nor does the child who grows out of night feedings at his own pace never outgrow them. Our child who was still coming in during the night at three and a half was, a year later, not only sleeping all through the night but was the last one to wake up in the morning.

HOW TO FEED YOUR BABY AT NIGHT

Nighttime feedings are no bother when mothers generally nurse in bed and fall asleep while doing so. "Horrors! What kind of a mother would admit to falling asleep while nursing her baby in bed?" These are common fears expressed by doctors, nurses, and acquaintances. These are fears that I also had with our first child. I heard about the advantages of nursing in bed, but I still couldn't overcome my fears of giving it a try so I'd sit in a chair for the night feedings. Oftentimes I was cold, and I was always tired. After fifteen or twenty minutes of nursing, I would take the baby off the breast even though she wanted to suck more in her sleep.

With our next baby, a nursing mother again encouraged me to try nursing the baby in bed. This was advice I still wouldn't accept. However, one afternoon I was so tired I fell asleep when nursing the baby and awoke three hours later to find the baby still at the breast. And to my surprise, she was safe and still sleeping and I was well rested. What a convenience!

16

I find that other nursing mothers are also reluctant to give it a try. They have these same acquired fears. Eventually some of them do give it a try, and then they begin to rave about the advantages of lying down to nurse the baby.

The fact that there is a natural instinct to protect your baby cannot be ignored; indeed, it's a good thing. Certainly, you must make sure your blankets or pillows are not near his face, or that your husband will not pull the blankets up over the baby. The baby may be dressed in a warm trundle bundle so that he can lie on top of the blankets. Other mothers tuck the baby right under the blankets, knowing he will turn his head completely away from the breast or up toward the head of the bed. Some mothers nurse with the baby in the center of the bed so that he will not fall off the bed, and they learn to offer the baby both breasts without changing the baby's position.

If the father is a light sleeper, the baby can sleep on the other side of his mother, near the side of the bed. When the baby is small, a chair can be placed at the side of the bed to prevent him from falling. Having a big, roomy bed, such as a king-size, is an asset to this type of program, although I have known parents who slept with their child in a regular double bed. When purchasing a larger bed consider the future savings from breastfeeding and from your not having to buy a baby crib.

Other arrangements have also been made. Some couples have slept on mattresses right on the floor with the baby's mattress right next to theirs. The baby can be nursed and then returned to your side on his own sleeping area. Even a foam cot or sleeping bag next to your bed will do. This same arrangement has been done with beds. The child's bed is placed next to the parents' bed on his mother's side. This close arrangement still allows the mother to nurse without restrictions; the child can be nursed as long as desired and still receive much cuddling in the process. The mother then has the option of returning the child to his bed later.

Some mothers find it difficult to nurse lying down at first, and some are never comfortable in any lying-down position. One mother who could not nurse lying down used a comfortable lounging chair for night feedings. Whichever way you choose, the important thing during the night is to be physically close enough to your child to sense his needs and to allow the child to nurse at his leisure without your getting tired.

Needless to say, if a mother has been drinking heavily or has been taking sleeping pills or is incapacitated in some way, it would not be a good practice to take the baby to bed with her that night. However, the point I would like to make is that the experience of nursing mothers shows that the baby who nurses in his mother's

bed runs no more risk of being smothered than he would with a
bottle and blanket in his own crib.

THE ADVANTAGES OF NIGHT FEEDINGS

It has already been said that the nursing mother finds that she
can satisfy her child's needs with little inconvenience or loss of
sleep. Being so close to her child, the mother can wake up temporarily at his first stir to offer him the breast. The child does not
have to stir and stir and then finally cry to get her attention as he
would if he were in a separate room. After offering the breast, the
mother then dozes back to sleep. This becomes so easy and natural
that often she could not say, if asked, how many times she nursed
during the night. Nursing a baby is one job you can do well in your
sleep.

Another advantage is the restfulness a mother can derive from
nursing in bed or lying down for naps. In fact, mothers who claim
to be the nervous type have noted the tranquilizing effect of
breastfeeding. Nursing can be a quieting and peaceful respite in
the midst of noise, anxieties, and irritations. This is why some
mothers will pick up their babies and nurse them on the rare night
that they cannot sleep. Nursing, besides putting baby to sleep, can
also put the mother to sleep. In addition, no matter how often or
how long the baby nurses during the night, the mother is generally
well rested and this restfulness is truly a big bonus for the entire
family. Mother can function better and enjoy her family; her good
disposition makes for a smoothly running day. She, likewise, is not
resentful—the baby did not keep her up all night, nor did her husband sleep through the night while she was up with the baby.
Indeed, the practice of night feedings as recommended in this
book may well improve family living.

What about burping? Do you have to get up to burp your baby?
Very frequently the baby who requires an occasional burping during the day will not require any burping at night. For a newborn
who does require burping, it is easy to place his head and shoulder
area up over your hip or stomach as you lie in bed.

What about changing diapers? I would recommend the use of
cloth cotton diapers (free of laundry soap) folded to allow for more
absorbency during the night. With the combination of breastfeeding and the use of cloth diapers, diaper rash is uncommon and a
baby can usually go through the night without a change.

A well-known advantage of breastfeeding is that the convenience eliminates a lot of decision making, and possibly arguing,
between husband and wife. They do not have to decide who shall

take care of the baby when it stirs or who will get up to warm the bottle. If the baby is already in their bed or next to it, the husband has another advantage—he doesn't have to get up even to bring the baby to bed.

Mothers have also written about how much they enjoyed these nightly snuggles with their baby. The cuddly, close relationship seems to have an emotional charge for the mother. But what's in it for father? Again, it comes down to a question of attitudes. Properly informed, he can see the advantages for the child, his wife, and himself. Over the years, I have heard from many couples that fathers truly enjoy this "bedtime" closeness, that they like waking up with their child at their side. For working parents— whether it be the father or the mother—it is one time that the baby can stay in touch with mom or dad after having had no contact with the parent during the day. I would strongly encourage working mothers to continue nursing so that 1) they can still enjoy this special closeness with their baby and 2) they can easily care for their baby during the night without feeling fatigued in the morning.

Some parents ask whether this practice will interfere with intimacy between husband and wife. Not if you have any imagination. At times of intimacy it is hardly necessary to bring the baby to bed until afterwards when you are ready to sleep. A couple who know their baby will awake soon may not choose to bring the baby to bed until later. Likewise, marital intimacies do not have to be confined to the bedroom.

Breastfeeding in bed has advantages for the baby, too. This is one time when he can nurse to full contentment in quiet, cozy surroundings. This is a time when his mother won't be interrupted, a time when he can use the breast to fulfill his sucking needs. It is known that babies at times will nurse on and off for

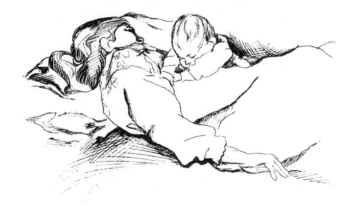

several hours while mother sleeps. This is common in the older breastfed child as well.

The most striking advantage for the baby is that this practice seems to play an important role in the child's emotional development because the baby keeps in **touch** with mother. The baby has a critical need for bodily contact with his mother; he **needs** to be caressed, cuddled, held, or just to be carried about with his mother. Some psychologists and writers today are quite concerned that most babies receive very little contact with their mother. This physical closeness with mother is all too often lacking, especially in our American culture.

An excellent article, "Of Babies, Beds and Teddy Bears" by Kenny and Schreiter,[1] documents the need for the infant to be in physical touch with his mother. Sleeping with one's baby is strongly encouraged, and support for this practice is given from psychological studies of other cultures. They show how sleeping together was once an American tradition until twin beds became quite popular in recent history. Good mothering is defined as much holding and cuddling of the baby, with emphasis given to sleeping together at night.

Ashley Montagu, in his book *Touching: The Human Significance of the Skin,*[2] demonstrates that the skin is the most important sensory organ we have and that the child needs to receive much skin stimulation from his mother in order to survive physically and emotionally. The sense of touch on the skin is the most alert sense during sleep, and therefore sleeping with babies is recommended at least for the entire first and second year. If the mother objects to sleeping with her child during the second year, he advises the mother to lie with her child at bedtime until he falls asleep. He uses other cultures as an example of that type of "touch" mothering which is so lacking in the American mother. Sleeping with the child is characteristic of the mother in these cultures where the child has lots of skin-to-skin contact with mother and, of course, where breastfeeding is common. If this contact at bedtime is not provided, Montagu says a cuddly toy may help but the child may resort to other activities, such as thumbsucking, rocking, and fondling of the genitals.

Dr. William Sears points out the merits of the family bed and offers advice for problem sleep situations in his excellent book, *Nighttime Parenting.*[3] The medical, emotional and other advantages are clearly demonstrated in his book. He finds that a baby likes to sleep for one, two or more years with his parents and that a child under three sleeps better when his sleep is shared with a parent or sibling.

I have often felt that there would be fewer cases of sudden infant death syndrome (SIDS) if parents slept with their babies but could never give a reason other than that the parents are much closer and in tune to their baby. Now it appears that the baby's closeness to his mother's body may be helpful for the newborn to develop the proper breathing pattern. I was pleased to hear of new research being done which supports what Dr. Margaret Ribble had claimed in her 1943 book, *The Rights of Infants*.[4] Ribble explained the various factors that can hamper a baby's breathing after birth and asked how a mother can facilitate her baby's breathing. The answer is to be found in sleeping with the baby. As she said, the mother furnishes the "stimulus which is necessary to bring important reflex mechanisms into action. It so happens that the baby's first response to her touch is respiratory. . .From being held, fondled, allowed to suck freely and frequently, the child receives reflex stimulation, which primes his breathing mechanisms into action and which finally enables the whole respiratory process to become organized under the control of his own nervous system." She noted that many women still fear that they will suffocate their baby, but she said the exact opposite is the truth. In her own words, the mother's contact as her child sleeps at her side "is a protection rather than a peril." After explaining the importance of the establishment of the respiratory system on the development of other areas of the body, she concluded: "The importance of mothering in helping the child to breathe at this time can hardly be stressed too greatly" and that "the quiet baby has to be watched with special care."

Very few SIDS cases are reported for totally breastfed babies, so breastfeeding must offer some protection against SIDS. There is also new evidence which supports what Dr. Ribble had claimed over forty-five years ago, and that is that sleeping with baby may prevent some of the cases of SIDS that strike one out of 500 American babies and is the leading killer of this nation's babies from one month to one year.[5] When napping with his son, Dr. James McKenna noticed that his baby's breathing pattern changed with his own. This led this anthropologist from the University of California at the Irvine Sleeping Center to monitor the breathing patterns and other vital signs of a parent and baby as they slept in separate rooms, as they slept in the same room, and as they slept in the same bed. Preliminary evidence indicates that the baby's breathing pattern followed the mother's when they slept together but not when they slept apart. With SIDS, babies stop breathing for no apparent reason and, according to him, ninety percent of these cases occur in babies younger than six months. McKenna explained that human breathing patterns change between the second and fourth months of life in preparation for speech. The doctor speculated that if parents slept with their babies SIDS might be prevented because infants would pick up cues that help their breathing systems mature. He said that sleeping with baby was very common in the past, but now it is considered bizarre. However, McKenna noted that sleeping separately "is a very recent and novel change in behavior."[6]

I'm also convinced that nature's plan is easier for both baby and the parents. When parents step in to hurry the process along, it's more trouble than it's worth, and in most cases, the baby suffers and is not as happy. True, these babies can turn out to be wonderful human beings as grown children and adults, but why make things complicated and make more work for yourselves as parents when there's an easier way?

Our last three children slept in bed with us at night for the first two years. This worked best for us. We didn't even begin to think of sleep separation until they were at least two years old. The transition period from the family bed was very gradual and took place over a period of another two years or more. In the beginning of the transition they would often start to sleep in our bed but occasionally begin to sleep in their bed or with a sibling. Toward the end they were likely to go to sleep in their bed. Usually they would end up in our bed during the early morning hours, but occasionally we noticed that they had slept through the night in their bed. Again, it was a very uneventful transition, much like child-led weaning. No fuss, no tears, so gradual that it almost happens unnoticed.

One of the most noted researchers in the area of mothering and lactation is Niles Newton, who has depicted the differences between bottle-feeding, what she calls token breastfeeding, and unrestricted breastfeeding. Token breastfeeding is typical of the American nursing mother today. Nursing is very limited; the baby receives little contact with mother; the baby sleeps in a different room because sleeping with the baby is considered dangerous; weaning occurs within a few weeks. However, with unrestricted breastfeeding, nursing is not restricted by rules; the child sleeps with or near his mother; the child has easy access to the breast day and night; no bottles are given to the baby and solids are begun only when baby is ready; the weaning process continues into early childhood. In addition, she notes that another characteristic of unrestricted nursing is a lengthy absence from menstrual periods.[7] Newton's description of unrestricted breastfeeding is exactly the type of mothering program I find necessary for natural spacing.

The mother who follows this pattern of unrestricted nursing experiences another aspect of the ecology of natural mothering. By taking care of the baby's needs for closeness, cuddling, and skin contact during the night, she also provides the opportunity for her baby to nurse as often as he pleases. A Chilean doctor confided to my husband that he encourages mothers to cuddle their babies between their breasts at night. This closeness provides stimulation through frequent nursing and helps prolong the natural infertility of breastfeeding.

To show the influence of sleeping with baby on the menstrual cycles, I would like to relate another true incident. The nursing mother experienced regular menstruation since childbirth. Her baby slept in another room, but that was to change when her husband went on a business trip for three months. When her husband left, she brought her nine month old baby to bed with her during the nights. She had no menstruation those three months during her husband's absence. The husband returned, her baby left her bed, and she soon noticed signs of returning fertility. I find this case extremely interesting since the only change in nursing behavior during those three months of amenorrhea was the nursing that took place during the night while the baby slept with his mother.

Mothers should do things for the right reasons, so I don't recommend night feedings or other aspects of natural mothering **just** to prolong amenorrhea. They should come out of the mother's realization that the nighttime closeness and nursing are good for both the baby and herself and that the extended amenorrhea is just a natural side effect.

If this approach were taken generally, then there would be fewer mothers who complain that to experience breastfeeding's natural infertility they would have to set the alarm, get up a couple times during the night to get the baby, and so on. I sympathize with these mothers because they have knowingly or unknowingly adopted the practices of a Western culture that goes strongly against the natural practices of unrestricted nursing. It is difficult to achieve the natural side effects of breastfeeding when part of the natural relationship is thwarted. Perhaps the question these mothers—and dads, too—should ask is, "If I were the baby, wouldn't I rather be close to my mother instead of all by myself? If I woke up during the night, wouldn't I rather be next to my mother who is ready to feed me rather than in a room with nobody else around?"

Yes, there are those who recommend the "tough" approach. "Make the baby realize that life is tough all over. Introduce it to the 'real world' as soon as possible." I disagree, and not only because the tough approach restricts the nursing pattern. It also incorporates a view of life that is very incomplete. In the real world, we soon realize that we can't make it on our own; we need a friend, someone who will bear with us even when we are less than perfect. So why not begin from the earliest months to let the baby know the friendship of his mother?

From everything said thus far, it should be evident that the mother who adopts this natural mothering approach isn't going to be thinking in terms of getting her baby to sleep through the night. She will let the baby set the pace. In fact, if the baby is an unusually heavy sleeper, she will want to encourage—not force—a nursing when she goes to bed and again when she first awakens. This relieves her breasts of excessive fullness and helps maintain a steady milk supply. It is also, according to some mothers, a most pleasant experience to nurse a sleepy baby at these times. The breast fullness seems to be nature's way of reminding the mother of her baby—and to be near her baby. It also helps the baby to get a regular intake of nourishment.

In summary, if a baby wakes up at night because of a need that can be fulfilled at the breast, there is no easier and better way for the family to get back to sleep than by letting the baby nurse at his mother's side in bed. This not only helps to satisfy the baby's nutritional and emotional needs, but satisfies the emotional needs of the mother. Not only is it restful for her, but she derives satisfaction in doing what is best for her baby and from having a contented and quiet baby as a result.

Sleeping with baby is an important practice for a mother to consider if she desires to space babies naturally—especially in our culture, where it's the custom to encourage babies to sleep through the night and to sleep apart from mother. These feedings help to maintain a more regular periodic feeding pattern throughout the twenty-four-hour day. They thus continue to provide frequent stimulation to the mother's breast and subsequently influence her body chemistry toward natural infertility.

References

1. James Kenny and Robert Schreiter, "Of Babies, Beds and Teddy Bears," *Marriage*, January 1971.
2. Ashley Montagu, *Touching: The Human Significance of the Skin* (New York: Columbia University Press, 1971).
3. William Sears, *Nighttime Parenting*, (New York: New American Library, 1987).
4. Margaret Ribble, *The Rights of Infants* (New York: Columbia University Press, 1943, 1965).
5. Lee Siegel, "Theory Links SIDS, Environment," *The Cincinnati Post*, May 28, 1985, p. C-1.
6. Sue MacDonald, "More on SIDS," *The Cincinnati Enquirer*, March 27, 1985, p. C-3.
7. Niles Newton, "Battle Between Breast and Bottle," *Psychology Today*, July 1972, p. 70.

4

Pacification of the Baby

Pacifiers have strongly influenced mothering today. They are of special interest here since they limit the amount of nursing and mothering at the breast. In fact, when regularly offered, the pacifier often receives more attention from the baby than the bottle or the breast.

We have already spoken of the role that the breast plays in pacifying the baby. It is also true that not only the breast but the mother's entire body plays an important role here as well. Her body is very adaptable. Her fingers can stroke and tease. Her knuckle or chin can act as a "pacifier" when the baby does not desire the breast. Her face and her voice offer expressions of love and happiness that tell the baby that he is someone very special. Her body offers motion and rhythm—two things babies love and which they receive when their mothers hold them, rock them, or carry them. The mother provides an "infant seat" for her baby when she sits and crosses one knee. Certain leg positions can form a cradle for her baby; when her legs move, baby is gently rocked. A good mother is needed, and no one can replace her. Sometimes her presence is all that is needed to change a baby's cries into smiles. Truly, a mother is the best pacifier for her baby.

I have been told that in former generations when breastfeeding was commonplace, some nursing mothers used various objects that served the same purposes as our rubber pacifiers. However, the present enormous popularity of the nipple-shaped pacifier seems to have started in the early 1950s.

WHY A PACIFIER?

The most obvious reason for offering the pacifier is to soothe and comfort the baby without nursing. Less obviously, it is also

25

used to pacify the parent who is thus spared the trouble of nursing or just holding the baby: parents tend to put the baby whose cries have been silenced by the pacifier back into the infant seat, crib, or playpen as soon as they can get away with doing so.

Some nursing mothers claim that they can't get along without the pacifier. Their babies are too fussy, or the mothers have too much milk and the baby wants to nurse on an empty breast, not a full one. Let's take a look at these reasons.

"THE BABY IS TOO FUSSY"

It can be expected that most babies will have an occasional fussy spell. This doesn't mean that it will happen every day, but it may happen several times a week. Some mothers may find that it seems a common occurrence in the early evening hours or when a baby is teething. It is always helpful to remember that eventually your baby will outgrow this fussiness. In addition, some babies will be alert and awake for a long period of time although they will not be fussy in an uncomfortable sense. Instead, they want lots of cuddling and holding or the presence of their mothers. Fortunately, there are ways to soothe a baby without resorting to the pacifier. After all, women got along without them for years!

Here are some suggestions:

1. Make sure the baby is neither too cold nor too warm; many mothers tend to overdress a baby.

2. Offer the breast, or see first if baby is interested by placing him in the nursing position.

3. Rock, hold, carry, walk, sway, dance, or sing to the baby. Rub or pat his back. Try lying down on your back and placing the baby on top of you; the movements of your chest may comfort him. Your husband can be a big help here when nursing isn't the answer.

4. Take a warm bath with the baby. Babies love to take baths with their mothers. There's more physical contact and security for the baby, it's easier and more fun for mother, and it has a relaxing effect on both. You may find that afterwards your baby will nurse into a deep sleep.

5. Weather permitting, take baby for a walk outdoors. Baby slings and back carriers are ideal for this type of activity. Some babies sleep well in the car, so if it's a weekend, maybe you and your husband would like to take a drive out in the country. For baby's safety, use a car seat in the back. At times when baby is

extremely fussy, you can sit next to him and lean over to nurse him if it's inconvenient for your husband to stop the car.

6. Offer the breast again. A baby may refuse the breast initially and yet welcome it only fifteen minutes later.

7. If your baby is continually fussy or colicky, review the La Leche League manual, *The Womanly Art of Breastfeeding*, for helpful suggestions or call a local La Leche League leader, if available, for support and helpful suggestions that have worked for other nursing mothers.

There may be a time when none of the above suggestions will help. I have had friends who had colicky babies, and they have remarked that the best thing to do was just continue the 100 percent nursing and give them lots of the physical contact all babies need. Their husband's help and support during this time was especially important to them. With most babies, however, the fussiness is brief, and normally a mother can find a more "natural" solution to baby's discomfort than using a pacifier. A mother who naps with her baby after lunch is also better disposed to handle any fussiness that occurs later in the day.

"I HAVE TOO MUCH MILK"

There will be times for most babies when it looks as if they are having difficulty handling the milk that comes from their mother's breast. The milk comes too fast, and the baby is inclined to fuss and pull away from the breast temporarily until the milk flow slows down. It is a situation more common for the baby in his early months; as he grows older, he will enjoy this ample supply. Other babies have satisfied their need for food but desire to nurse more. What they want is an empty breast, not one full of milk; so they react quite strongly against the breast that is full.

There really isn't any problem in the first situation. The occasional time that this happens the mother can allow for more burping or wait until the "let-down" feeling—which is what causes the milk to come out so fast—has been completed. But don't wait if baby is crying, please. If baby is hungry, he'll be anxious to get back on the breast. So let him; if it's too much for him to handle again, he'll pull off and keep trying. If, however, this situation occurs at almost every feeding, you might find some of these ideas helpful.

1. Try a different nursing position, such as lying down. At night mothers seldom have this problem when sleeping with baby.

2. Try offering the breast so that the spray angles off to the side

or top of the baby's mouth and not directly toward the back of his throat.

3. Offer only one breast at a feeding. This way the baby can satisfy his other sucking needs toward the end of the feeding on a breast that isn't full of milk. A small infant can receive plenty of milk from one breast at a feeding, especially when the supply is ample. At the next feeding offer the other breast.

4. The mother who has a huge supply for a month or two after childbirth might offer the same breast for approximately a two-hour period. In other words, she would feed the baby, let's say, at 9:00 a.m. Then, if an hour later the baby wanted to nurse again, the mother would offer the same breast she offered at 9:00. During the next two-hour period she would offer the other breast. This feeding pattern could be used until the milk supply settled and the baby could handle it better.

Normally, one-breast feedings with unrestricted and frequent nursing do not present any problems. However, since in using this method there is an increased risk of engorgement or a plugged duct with an abundant supply of milk, the mother should be observant. If a breast becomes too full and drippy, she can express the excess milk by hand. If a tender spot is felt on the breast, she can let the baby suck on that breast as much as possible to keep it empty (plus additional hand expression during a let-down, if necessary), and usually the tenderness will disappear as quickly as it appeared.

Proper management of an overabundant milk supply may be a factor in the maintenance of infertility. For example, one mother wrote that she had so much milk that her four-month-old did not have to suckle; her milk supply was so ample that it just flowed into his mouth. She also felt that this was why she had menstruated since childbirth. A few other mothers have also felt that "an over-ample supply" might have been the cause of an early return of menstruation following childbirth. The above practices designed to increase the amount of actual suckling may help in these cases too.

"WE WANT TO AVOID THUMB-SUCKING"

Normally many parents have another purpose in mind besides pacifying when they offer the pacifier regularly to their babies. They want to avoid thumb-sucking and, possibly, any future orthodontic expenses. Dentists hold varying opinions on the matter. In 1961 an orthodontist at the University of California School of Dentistry in San Francisco taught my class that (1) the young child should be encouraged to suck his thumb if he desires and that parents should not discourage this habit until after the child is four years old; (2) thumb-sucking will cause no harm to the permanent set of teeth if the child sucks up until four years of age; (3) the child's sucking needs are best satisfied at an early age when the child is allowed to nurse as much as he desires; and (4) breastfeeding satisfies this need best. Many dentists now support the view that thumb-sucking does the child no harm until he is five or six years old, or until the time when his baby teeth begin to loosen. A few dentists will advocate "no thumb-sucking" because they feel that it will cause harm to the permanent set of teeth. Interestingly, some of these dentists also advocate "no pacifiers," since they feel that the prolonged use of either habit causes the same problems.

But no matter what view is held by a particular dentist or orthodontist, almost all are in agreement that suckling at the breast is better than sucking at bottles and pacifiers from the point of view of dental care. First, breastfeeding prevents tongue thrusting. Tongue thrusting develops in an infant who pushes his tongue forward to slow down the fast flow of milk from a bottle and prevent the flooding of milk at the back of the throat. I was told in dental school that I had a slight tongue thrusting swallow, but not enough to cause any problems. I was a bottle baby. Severe tongue thrusting, however, can interfere with speech and teeth alignment.

Mr. Daniel Garliner, a speech specialist, who has lectured extensively to medical, dental and orthodontic groups in various parts of the United States and Canada, claims that we swallow 2,000 times a day! Thus one can see that if a child swallows incorrectly, his parents could be paying for speech therapy and dental correction. How do we prevent a deviate swallow or tongue thrusting in our children? Breastfeeding is the answer. As Garliner says: Mother Nature "had designed the nursing act to be a forerunner of the speech act. Mothers were designed to nurse babies. It was imperative that the muscles of swallowing would receive sufficient exercises," so that "the infant would develop strong oral muscles." When the mother resorts to bottles and enlarged holes in the rubber nipple for speedy feedings, the fluid comes so quickly toward the back of his throat that the child has to protect himself. His only protection is his tongue which the baby uses to push forward. Once he learns this, a deviate swallow has developed.[1]

In the breastfeeding act, the baby has control of 1) "the length of the nipple, 2) the flow from the nipple, and 3) the flexibility of the nipple substance," according to Garliner in his book *Swallow Right—Or Else*. With artificial feeding, the baby loses the control in these three areas. "There is no question that breastfeeding is the most desirable situation for the infant in terms of muscle development," and failure to provide a substitute for nature's system, said Garliner, has led to "weakened facial musculature, more dental malocclusions, and speech defects."[2]

The stronger suckling that breastfeeding requires involves a muscular action that promotes the proper growth and development of the jaw, bones, and muscular tissues of the entire face. Studies show that the presence of long-term nursing tends to decrease the need for orthodontic work. Breastfeeding is the first step in preventive orthodontics. Of course, orthodontic problems may arise from other factors that cannot be controlled by healthy sucking habits.

Both my husband and I were typical bottle-fed babies and we both required extensive orthodontic work as youngsters. None of our children, however, required any orthodontic work, a rare experience for a family in a neighborhood full of braces.

In studying the histories of 9,698 children, researchers at the Johns Hopkins School of Public Health found "that children bottle-fed or breastfed for less than a year reported misaligned teeth 40 percent more often than children breastfed for more than one year. . .But those breastfed for three months or less and those who continued to suck a finger had the highest risk of crooked teeth." They concluded that breastfeeding contributes to straighter teeth because "it leads to different growth patterns in the mouth than those in bottle-fed babies."[3]

The relationship between the use of the bottle as a pacifier and tooth decay has also been highlighted in the daily press and by dental organizations. What happens when the bottle is used as a pacifier is that the baby takes a couple of sucks and then swallows, but a little of the bottle's contents still seeps into the mouth and touches the teeth. The teeth are actually bathed or surrounded by the milk or juice from the bottle. An acquaintance of ours had this unpleasant experience to the tune of three hundred dollars' worth of dental work that had to be done on her eighteen-month-old, bottle-pacified child. The child needed his four front teeth capped and required both hospitalization and the service of an anesthesiologist. The dentist explained that this decay was due to the lactic acid in the cow's milk used in the bottle-pacifier.

Breastfeeding, especially lying-down nursing, is often accused of causing this decay termed "nursing bottle syndrome." However, the act of obtaining milk when breastfeeding is completely different. The baby has to work for his milk and then swallows. If baby falls asleep at the breast, there is no milk that pools around the teeth when he is not nursing. This important fact has been proven by a detailed study where combined pictures of motion pictures and radiography of breastfeeding babies showed that no milk accumulates in the mouth during nursing or after its cessation.[4] Dr. Louis M. Abbey, a professor of oral pathology at the Virginia Commonwealth University School of Denistry, has studied the available literature on this subject and finds there is no convincing evidence which implicates the practice of unrestricted breastfeeding as a cause of early caries in infants.[5]

It must be remembered that dental decay is not caused by a single factor. The mother's diet and even her health during pregnancy can affect the formation of her child's teeth; the hygiene of her baby's teeth and his diet also influence the health of baby's teeth. For good dental hygiene, you can clean your child's teeth several times a day even when breastfeeding and avoid giving your older baby sweets or highly refined foods such as the popular soda crackers that can convert readily to sugar. Remember that dried fruits such as raisins are bad for teeth; when taken, you should follow up with a good brushing and even a slim carrot or celery stick. Avoid honey during your child's first year to avoid botulism. It can be used after the child's first birthday but should be followed up with a good cleaning by the parent. This was not meant to be a discussion on oral hygiene but to show you that other factors come into play when discussing dental decay. In addition, our dentist claims the dental decay rate has been cut drastically since Cincinnati added fluoride to the drinking water. He is seeing many more youngsters today who are cavity-free.

On the other hand, we know that some breastfed babies do develop decay on their front teeth. In these situations, it is usually best to be conservative with a "wait and see" attitude and continue to keep these teeth well cleaned. I nursed four of our children with lying-down nursing. Two had no sign of front tooth decay and two did: one major and one very minor. With the major case (our fourth child), I had a fever during the pregnancy that could have affected the developing tooth buds. We were thankful for a dentist who from his experience with his own children preferred the conservative approach. Finally, prior to kindergarten one of her laterals was bothering her, and he recommended a pediatric oral surgeon. Since the other lateral tooth was very similar in appearance, she had both removed; the experience was such a pleasant one that she wanted to go back to have her central incisors, which were quite ugly, removed. Never were we so happy to see those teeth loosen and beautiful new teeth replace them. We also continued the breastfeeding relationship as our dentist never told me to wean. I also appreciate the fact that he did not insist on hospitalization and treatment at such an early age. By waiting, we treated only what was necessary; we limited ourselves to an office visit; when the laterals were removed, she was older and the surgery was not traumatic. In addition, the selection of the right practitioner made the surgery go smoothly; one of the reasons for this was that the parent was allowed to stay until the child was asleep. I might add that this child is now in her mid-teens and hasn't had a cavity for a half dozen years as of this writing. My advice to mothers who find themselves in similar situations is to continue the nursing as previously, but consult several dentists, if that's what it takes, before you find one who is good with children and tends to take the conservative approach. When we moved to Cincinnati, I went to three dentists for regular dental care before I found one who I felt would be good with children.

PACIFIER PROBLEMS

Pacifiers may be dangerous objects. Some tend to break into pieces which can cut or choke a baby. Pacifiers are also a ready source of all sorts of germs, dirt, and other things. An acquaintance from Brazil told me that the mothers all nursed their children but that they also used bottles and pacifiers. He then spoke of the poor sanitation, and he was especially concerned about the various types of worms the child could ingest by sucking on a dirty pacifier. Government regulation can reduce design and manufacturing problems but obviously can do nothing about hygiene.

Pacifiers may create problems instead of solving them for the nursing mother. These difficulties were described in the La Leche League *Leaven* (May-June 1972) by a counseling mother.

It happened again, and I am finally moved to write. A mother called with a six-month-old baby on a nursing strike. Among other things I asked if she used a pacifier with her baby. I was almost sure the answer would be "yes," and it was. This is getting to be one of my routine counseling questions. When a mother with a one-month-old calls because her baby isn't gaining weight, or a mother calls because her three-month-old seems to be going through a growth spurt but will only nurse while the milk flows freely, nine times out of ten these babies suck long and frequently on pacifiers.

Perhaps I am so aware of this because heavy pacifier use was one of the downfalls in nursing our firstborn. He, too, nursed only for milk and got his main comfort from the pacifier. He would never nurse at length to build up a greater supply; during growth spurts I added extra solid food. By five months the nursing just petered out.

Even if the situation never gets this drastic, isn't one of the joys of nursing found in being your own baby's "pacifier"? To be able to soothe your little one at the breast when he needs this comforting form of love is one of the nicest inherent advantages of breastfeeding.

The baby can fill up in a few minutes when at the breast, but there are many times, especially when tired, that he will need to be pacified at the breast. You can see how soothing the breast is when you allow your baby to remain there. The breast may even bring comfort to a bottle-fed baby. We had one acquaintance tell us of their adopted baby who was extremely fussy and nothing worked in her efforts to quiet him down. She had no intentions of nursing this baby, but out of frustration she offered the breast. To her surprise, it worked. It was at these difficult times that she used the breast to soothe her baby.

The absence of pacifiers may be crucial in the maintenance of natural infertility. Nature provided the baby with his mother's breast and with his own fingers for satisfying his sucking needs. Artificial devices replace nature's products—and, as we have seen, the absence of natural baby care usually means the absence or shortening of natural child spacing. The two go together.

The following two stories show that total nutritional breastfeeding does not assure the breastfeeding infertility, as both mothers nursed totally for a considerable length of time and yet both experienced menstrual periods while doing so. However, their babies did use the pacifier regularly.

One mother had two periods by the time she was five months postpartum and totally nursing. She told me this while her second child was cradled in her arms, sucking on a pacifier. We began to talk about pacifiers and how the babies are taught to suck on them instead of the breast; this was then related to the importance of the sucking act for the natural suppression of fertility. She said she had nursed her first baby although not totally. Yet with him, up to the age of her present five-month-old, she had not menstruated—and she never gave her first baby a pacifier.

Another friend, who nursed her baby for seven months before introducing solids, experienced regular periods after childbirth. She nursed her baby every three and a half to four hours and offered him a pacifier so she "wouldn't have to nurse the baby all the time." Interestingly enough, this mother, after having several periods, then missed two periods during the time that she was expressing milk for another baby in addition to feeding her own. Maybe this extra stimulation suppressed her menses, for they resumed after she no longer expressed the extra milk for the other baby and was once again only providing for her own.

Does the pacifier make the difference? This is an interesting question, since the nursing, when limited to the baby's nutritional needs, does not seem to be effective in holding back menstruation in many cases. If the babies in the above stories had been pacified as well as fed at the breast, maybe the additional suckling might have been sufficient to provide breastfeeding's normal infertility.

THUMB-SUCKING

The absence of pacifiers automatically leads to the subject of thumb-sucking, a subject which deserves more consideration and study with respect to mothering. Dr. James Clark Moloney, writing in *Child and Family* magazine,[6] discussed pathological thumb-sucking and attempted to show that the baby who sucks his thumb may be "mothering" himself; the thumb may become a substitute for the mother's breast and body. He explained how mother-body contact and free access to the breast provide satisfaction and reassurance to the infant, and how such an infant has no need for a substitute. Noting other cultures, he told of the Okinawan mother who places her baby at breast immediately after birth and continues to remain in close touch with him. The child is carried on his mother's back, and she caresses and cuddles him. The child sleeps on a mat with his parents. He is allowed to creep and crawl and explore on his own, yet he knows he can return to his mother's side any time he desires. The baby is so closely related to his mother that she senses his needs before he cries. He pointed out that unfortunately many American mothers tend to minister to their infants and then set them aside and leave them, treating them in what he called an undesirable arm's-length manner. Our culture tends to produce thumb-suckers since maternal intimacy is lacking.

It is obvious that excessive thumb-sucking would have the same effect as a pacifier on the natural spacing processes in some cases, so some mothers have felt very strongly that the baby should not suck his thumb or fingers at all. I cannot be so strong about this issue. Some babies will suck their fingers often in spite of frequent nursing and close contact with mother. Babies may want to suck temporarily when uncomfortable—during a burping session or when teething, for example—and they will begin to suck upon awakening from their sleep as hunger develops. This sucking signals a need to his mother who can offer the breast before he is fully awake and probably crying. Rather obviously, she will have to be physically close to him to notice such needs.

Physical closeness makes the mother more aware of her child's needs—so much so that it will normally be a requirement for natural spacing. Natural mothering, with its physical mother-baby closeness and unrestricted nursing, does not come easily in our society. With little outside support, most of us have learned the "art of mothering" through caring for two, three, or even seven babies. I admire and almost envy the young mother who has all this information before the birth of her first child. She can adopt this type of mothering right away and receive the joys that come from it in her first effort. Some of us have felt that we did a good job of mothering only to discover that with our next child we were still doing things a bit differently. We mature and learn with each child. The difference may be slight, but it appears to be enough to eliminate the thumb-sucking in some cases. Table I shows how three children were raised, each a little differently, by one mother.

May I quote the mother's remarks about thumb-sucking?

[Our first child] started sucking his fingers fairly early but I don't remember exactly when. He spontaneously gave this up when he was about four and a half years old or a little more. [Our second child] started sucking her thumb before she was a year old and became quite an inveterate thumb-sucker. At four and a half she still sucks it a lot, chiefly at night or when tired or upset. I think our children must have a tremendous sucking need, and although I was more free in nursing this second child, and she in fact nursed a lot more than "average," it was obviously not enough to prevent the thumb-sucking. [Our third child] is by far the most independent of our three, and the only one who has never sucked thumb or fingers. I have the feeling that if it weren't for so much nursing she would definitely have been a thumb-sucker. Occasionally I have seen her put her thumb in her mouth and start to half-suck, and then I would always pick her up for a nursing.

Her experiences tend to show a relationship between thumb-sucking and the amount of nursing and physical contact with mother. It is interesting to note that as this mother gradually developed a more natural mothering style with each child, her length of infertility after childbirth increased.

It is not my intention to leave the impression that anything more than the tiniest bit of thumb-sucking will destroy the ecological balance. From my own experience, and from that of some other mothers, it is evident that a mother who adopts the natural mothering style may still have a baby who sucks his fingers or thumbs quite a bit without the mother having an early return of fertility. It is likewise true that some thumb-suckers with frequent unrestricted nursing may stop sucking on their hands at a later date and use only the breast for pacification.

Table I: Different Styles of Mothering and Their Effects on Fertility

	CHILD #1	CHILD #2	CHILD #3
PACIFIER	For only 3 months	None	None
BOTTLE	Gave 72 ounces during early postpartum weeks; mother had serious breast infections	None	None
SOLIDS BEGUN	At 6 months; with spoon	At 6 months; with spoon	At 9 months; with finger foods
CUP BEGUN	At 9 months; mother offered cup	After one year; on his own	After one year; on his own
NURSING COMPLETED	At 16 months	At 27 months	Still nursing often at 28 months
NIGHT FEEDINGS	First 6 months; then baby slept through	First 6 months; then baby slept through	Still nurses at night at 28 months
SLEEPING ARRANGEMENT AT NIGHT	In the crib	Mother nursed baby in bed but returned to crib	In parents' bed
PERIODS RESUMED	At 12 months postpartum	At 18 months postpartum	Never did; mother encouraged reduced nursings to achieve pregnancy, which occurred 27 months postpartum
THUMB-SUCKING	3 months to 4-1/2 years	From 1 year to more than 4-1/2 years	Absent

The point I am emphasizing, however, is that mothering practices in which the mother takes care of the nutritional and emotional sucking needs of the infant are those which reinforce the mother-baby ecology and tend to postpone the return of fertility and menstruation. The mother who adopts the philosophy of physical closeness and who has her baby physically near her at night as well as during the day is in a position to recognize the various sucking needs of her infant. When she satisfies these needs at the breast, she cooperates with the natural pattern. Offering the breast when she notices her baby sucking his thumb or fingers not only provides some milk and emotional comfort and reinforces the ecological relationship; it also may reduce or prevent a habit of thumb-sucking from birth or at a later date. Some of my correspondents have been quite emphatic on this whole subject, and some have stated their plans to offer the breast more with a future child when they see him sucking his thumb. The current reader has the choice and can benefit from our accumulated experience. It must be remembered, however, that some babies will at times prefer their fingers to the breast.

OTHER SOOTHERS

The child-care industry has come up with any number of things that can be used as mother substitutes. Used to excess, they not only interfere with the mother-baby ecology of breastfeeding and natural infertility; they can also hinder his development[7] and even lead to death from "unknown causes." For example, hospitals have found that infants need tender, loving care and that infants deprived of this care and physical contact will wither and not develop normally. We have heard the story of an orphanage where, some time ago, infants, kept in cribs, were given adequate nutrition and sanitation but where there was still a high rate of unexplained sickness and subnormal progress and development—except for the babies right near the door. Finally it was realized that the babies near the door were getting little bits of extra attention from nurses and maids as they came in and out of the door—patting them on the head, speaking to them, and so forth. From such examples we can see that even the crib or a playpen can be used in such a way that it becomes a prison instead of just a temporary protection against falling or getting hurt in some way.

I have heard of mothers who almost worshiped the infant seat. No one was permitted to pick up the baby, so a piece of plastic became its habitual home. Perhaps one of the devices that is most easy to use to excess is the spring-wound swing. Just place the baby in the seat, wind it up, and baby may be content, almost hypnotically so, for literally hours. One former neighbor bragged about the fact that her baby ate and slept in such a swing. I don't think it requires much imagination to see how such baby-care practices may result in greatly reduced mother-baby contacts and breastfeeding, thus upsetting the ecology of breastfeeding and natural infertility.

Again, one's attitudes change. With our first baby we thought a playpen was an absolute necessity, but we rarely used it. We lost it in a move and never replaced it. Many devices are temporarily helpful to the mother, and even temporarily enjoyable to the baby. However, often their use can be called into question if the mother tends to rely on them.

The device I found most helpful is the back carrier. I used the same carrier for five children and found it invaluable. For newborns and small babies under six months old, a cloth carrier is recommended so that the baby can be carried on mother's front. A cloth carrier as described in my reference note[8] can be made very inexpensively and it provides the same support as similar cloth baby carriers I've seen advertised in the $30-$45 range (1989 dollars). In contrast with other devices, the baby carrier is not a mother substitute but actually helps to provide the same type of closeness given by similar carriers among the more nature-oriented peoples of the world.

References

1. Daniel Garliner, *Your Swallow: An Aid to Dental Health* (The Gulf Building, Suite 715, 95 Merrick Way, Coral Gables, FL), six page pamphlet.
2. Garliner, *Swallow Right—Or Else* (St. Louis: Warren H. Green, 1979.)
3. "Breastfeeding Linked to Straighter Teeth," *The New York Times*, June 2, 1987.
4. G.M. Ardran et al., "A Cineradiographic Study of Breastfeeding," *Br. J. Radiol.* 31(March 1958)156.
5. Louis M. Abbey, "Is Breastfeeding a Likely Cause of Dental Caries in Young Children?" *JADA* 98(January 1979)21.
6. James Clark Moloney, "Thumb-sucking," *Child and Family*, Summer 1967.
7. Bonnie Prudden, *Is Your Child Really Fit?* (New York: Harper & Row, 1956).
8. Baby carriers are available at department stores, baby stores, and camping-outfitting stores. A homemade front sling for the baby is easy to make, and no sewing is required. Take 2-1/2 yards of fabric 36 inches wide and tie the ends together in a double knot. Wear it as a sling over one shoulder and across your chest with the knot in back, and you can put it on or remove it without untying the knot. Baby will fit securely in front, as the material tucks in tightly around his buttocks (his legs hang free) and offers support for his head. Extra material gathered around the baby's shoulders can be pulled up over his head to provide protection on an extremely windy or sunny day.
A sturdy denim baby carrier with padded straps is also available through the Couple to Couple League. See mini-catalog at back of book.

5

The Frequency Factor

Frequent unrestricted nursing is a common occurrence among mothers who follow the type of natural mothering described in this book. As I have mentioned before, it's this frequency which prolongs natural infertility following childbirth. The conditions leading to frequent nursing which we have not discussed yet are the absence of any feeding schedules and the physical closeness of mother and baby. The oneness of the mother-baby relationship, sometimes called traditional inseparability, is crucial when following the natural mothering program and will be covered in the following chapter.

A mother must learn to ignore advice about schedules—unless, of course, there is a serious medical reason for them. Today a nursing mother may be told that at such-and-such-a-time every day she will be feeding her baby and that by a certain age she will be feeding her baby only three or four times during the day. She might be told to nurse at least twenty minutes on each side. While in the hospital she may be told to nurse only five minutes on each side and that's all! One friend told me that she was even told when she could bathe the baby, put it to sleep, and play with him. Obviously, such schedules are geared for adults and not babies. No consideration is given to the true needs of the baby— whether or not the baby is hungry or full, tired or sociable, dirty or clean.

The popular four-hour schedule is not popular with breastfed babies. Many breastfed babies will nurse several times during that amount of time. On occasion you may find yourself nursing your baby quite often, or even within the same hour. This shouldn't surprise us. After all, we adults often get up from the table only to find ourselves snacking an hour later or drinking between meals.

Many parents feel that a baby should be put on a schedule so he will not manipulate his parents. It is feared that he will control the mother unless she controls him. He can even ruin family life and be a threat to a good marriage unless he is strictly scheduled and shown his place in the home! The emphasis here is on power rather than love. A baby has no complex ideas about controlling anyone. Nor can a baby and his needs be blamed for a deteriorating marital relationship. On the contrary, the sight of one's spouse going out of his or her way to take care of the baby's needs can be a source of renewed pride, but this is not to say that a baby is a cure for a poor marriage relationship. A baby has no plan for making people happy or unhappy.

Schedules simply have no place in natural mothering. In bottle-feeding, they serve the purpose of keeping babies from being starved by some mothers and overstuffed by others. However, in nature's baby-care plan, mother and baby are always together, and the mother very quickly senses her baby's nursing needs. This can contribute to the mother's self-esteem as she realizes her unique importance for her baby; it can also help develop her capacity for self-giving as she responds to his needs instead of scheduling him to fit her convenience.

Nursing mothers generally comment that things run more smoothly once they accept the more frequent feedings and forget the clock— and this applies even when the baby is older. In brief, rules are confusing because the schedule says one thing and the baby is telling mother something else. Mothering and breast-feeding are usually easier for both mother and baby when the mother takes her cues from the baby and learns to relax with this flexibility.

From the preceding paragraph it should be clear why schedules will most likely upset the breastfeeding baby-spacing ecology. The baby who is allowed to develop under the natural mothering program may be nursing every couple of hours during the day, sometimes even more frequently, thus giving his mother the frequent suckling stimulation that is necessary for her fertility to remain at rest.

Since the first writing of this book in 1967-68, more attention has been given to frequent nursing episodes and their effect upon lactation amenorrhea. Dr. Peter W. Howie, working with a research team in Edinburgh, Scotland, asked why some nursing mothers ovulated much later than other nursing mothers. The answer was related to the amount of suckling frequency. Those nursing mothers who ovulated early nursed the least amount during the day, reduced the nursing times fastest, introduced other foods quickly and gave up night feedings rapidly. On the other hand, the nursing mothers who suppressed ovulation for a longer period of time continued to give night feedings, nursed oftener, introduced other foods slowly, and reduced their nursing times gradually. Howie concluded that "the effectiveness of suckling as an inhibitor of ovulation is certainly dependent upon breastfeeding practice. The resumption of ovulation may be dependent upon other factors as well, but certainly we would suggest that suckling is a major variable, if not **the** major variable in the control of postpartum ovulation and fertility."[1]

Howie and his associates centered their work around the introduction of solids and the absence of night feedings, practices they felt undermined the amount and frequency of suckling and led to the return of ovarian activity. A contemporary American study provided the same results, that "night nursing after supplementation was a major factor in post-supplementation duration of amenorrhea."[2] In other words, among all nursing mothers who had introduced other foods, the most important practice in delaying a return of their periods after supplementation was nursing during the night. Those mothers who introduced other foods later and who night-nursed for at least one hour once supplementation was begun remained amenorrheic for six to ten months longer than those mothers who supplemented early and who reduced night feeds.

The effects of the breastfeeding frequency factor upon fertility were also studied by James Wood, research scientist at the University of Michigan's Population Studies Center; his subjects were a New Guinea people, the Gainj, where breastfeeding episodes were short and frequent. The child is fed on demand day and night with the nursling always sleeping with his mother. Solids are begun at about nine to twelve months of age with complete wean-

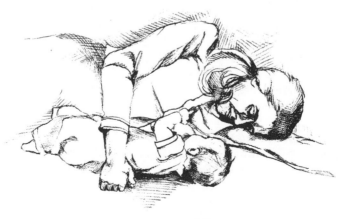

ing occurring at or near the child's third birthday. "The first solid foods given to the child (starchy tubers, bananas, papayas) are comparatively poor in nutrition so that breast milk remains the only reliable source of high quality protein and fat in the child's diet well into the second or even third year of life."

The demographic picture demonstrates the value of breastfeeding in this group where neither contraception nor abortion are practiced. The researchers explained that if these Gainj women abandoned breastfeeding, they would reduce their mean birth interval from 44 months to about 21 months, and the number of live births would more than double per woman from 4.3 to 9.2. As the researchers concluded, "the reproductive consequences of breastfeeding in this population are profound."

In this study, the frequency and intervals of the nursings were recorded, and breastfeeding for the Gainj mothers was characterized by frequent suckling and short suckling intervals. With their infants, these women averaged 24 minute intervals; with their three-year-olds, they averaged about 80 minutes between nursings; the reduction in suckling frequency occurred very slowly. The research team concluded: "The finding that suckling frequency is high and changes only slowly over time appears to be of special importance in explaining the prolonged contraceptive effect of breastfeeding in this population."[3]

The effect of frequent suckling was also observed among the !Kung tribe of the Kalahari Desert in southern Africa where the mothering and breastfeeding frequency patterns were similar to the Gainj people. (The ! in !Kung represents a tongue clucking sound.) !Kung women were conceiving on the average of 35 months postpartum, thus allowing almost four years between the birth of babies. It was also observed among these non-contracepting people that the little one remained physically close to his mother day and night during the first two years. Researchers Konner and Worthman concluded that the frequency factor was the likely key to the child spacing of these people—nursings of a few minutes duration occurring several times an hour.[4]

Nursing one's baby several times during the hour seems to be the norm, according to Dr. R. V. Short. He referred to two groups of hunter-gatherers: the !Kung tribe just mentioned and another in Papua, New Guinea, where mothers also nurse frequently. He thinks that "the biochemical composition of human milk, which is low in fat, protein and dry matter" fits into the need for frequent suckling. While "this high frequency of suckling may seem abnormal at first," Dr. Short holds that it is probably nature's norm. Even the chimps and the gorillas (the human species' closest relatives) suckle several times an hour in the wild, sleep with their babies, and have birth intervals of four or five years—similar to the two above mentioned primitive tribes. Dr. Short credits the frequent suckling stimulus as "the crucial factor in causing the contraceptive effect" of breastfeeding.[5]

Does this information alter our thinking and help us to see frequent suckling as a normal occurrence—even a desirable goal? How often does it happen that a mother who severely limits suckling at the breast feels a need to supplement her milk or finds that her baby is not gaining well or appears to be hungry a major part of the time? Unfortunately nursing only three to five times a day is seen as a very desirable goal among many nursing mothers, and frequent suckling is looked upon as a negative and undesirable practice.

Nursing is especially frowned upon in public places. As a result, many American mothers feel compelled to express milk in a bottle for use away from home. Mothers have noticed a return of menstruation after visiting relatives over the holidays. They find themselves in an environment unfavorable towards breastfeeding and they reduce their nursings considerably. Our society discourages public nursing or nursing outside the family circle so that most people have not seen a baby at the breast. If they have seen a baby nurse, most likely the baby was their brother or sister or a very close friend's or relative's.

A mother has to be determined to follow ecological breastfeeding with unrestricted nursing in a society where this type of breastfeeding is often unwelcome. She can learn how to nurse comfortably in various social situations so the nursings need not be reduced or eliminated. And as her baby continues to nurse frequently with age, she will learn to be comfortable with this continued pattern as well. The studies I quoted from reinforce what I have learned from personal experience and from other nursing mothers, namely, that with long-term nursing the frequency continues for an extended time and gradually diminishes toward the time of complete weaning. Usually the frequency of nursing is such that a mother hardly notices any changes in the frequency because the change is so gradual. But she will notice changes toward the end of the breastfeeding relationship.

It may sound as if all a mother does is nurse her baby without doing anything else. This is a false picture, although I have heard a few nursing mothers relate how their babies required constant nursing. This is unusual though and not the norm. With ecological breastfeeding, the baby nurses frequently but the feedings are brief. The times that the feedings are long usually occur when the baby is upset or hurt—which usually isn't often— and when he is tired prior to falling asleep. The mother can reassure herself from the research and the experience of other nursing mothers that her baby's frequent nursing pattern is normal, is part of God's plan for mother and child with its many benefits, and is the type of breast-feeding associated with extended postpartum infertility.

References

1. P.W. Howie, "Synopsis of Research on Breastfeeding and Fertility," paper presented at the Fourth National and International Symposium on Natural Family Planning, November 1985. Published in *Breastfeeding and Natural Family Planning*, ed. Mary Shivanandan (Bethesda: KM Associates, 1986).

2. M. Elias, et al., "Nursing Practices and Lactation Amenorrhea," *Journal of Biosocial Science* 18:1(January 1986)1.

3. James W. Wood, et al., "Lactation and Birth Spacing in Highland New Guinea," *Journal of Biosocial Science*, Suppl., 9(1985)159.

4. Melvin Konner and Carol Worthman, "Nursing frequency, gonadal function, and birth spacing among !Kung hunter-gatherers," *Science* 207(Feb. 15, 1980)788.

5. R.V. Short, "Breast Feeding", *Scientific American*, 250(April 1984)35.

6

Mother and Baby as One

This chapter should make it clear that the purpose of this book is not to encourage ecological breastfeeding **just** to have an extended time of natural infertility. Rather, the purposes of this book are first to help mothers give their babies the best start in life and then to explain how the practice of natural mothering normally results in extended postpartum infertility. Chapter Ten reviews some of the physiological reasons for calling ecological breastfeeding the best start; this chapter looks at psychological reasons.

The importance of the good start in life is emphasized by Dr. Burton White, director of the Parent Education Center in Newton, Massachusetts, who has spent years researching what causes competent people to get that way:

On the basis of years of research, I am totally convinced that the first priority with respect to helping each child to reach his maximum level of competence is to do the best possible job in structuring his experience and opportunities during the first three years of life.[1]

My research leads me to believe that what I'm calling "natural mothering" is at the heart of providing that best experience. Ecological breastfeeding is part of a child-centered way of baby care. As such, it runs counter to the typical American culture which is not child-centered but, rather, is adapted to providing immediate convenience to parents. I stress the idea of **immediate** convenience because it may well be that the short-term conveniences connected with early child care contribute to problems later on. For example, if properly breastfed babies have only one-tenth as many allergy problems as bottle-fed babies, has the overall "convenience" of the bottle been worth it? Or, if women who have both bottle-fed and breastfed tell me, as they have, that they have somehow developed a different, better, warmer relationship with their breastfed babies, what might this mean in terms of the long-term relationship between mother and child?

Two indications of an adult-centered baby care are the attitudes and practices with regard to schedules and baby-sitters. Schedules, which we have already discussed, are obviously for adult convenience, and the presence of baby-sitters means that mother and baby are being separated, possibly for long periods of time—thus upsetting the breastfeeding-child spacing ecology. If a couple say that this baby isn't going to change in any way their active social life, it could hardly be more obvious that their whole way of life, including baby care, is centered around themselves as on-the-go adults. Such an attitude would most likely run into direct conflict with the baby-centered program that is essential for the ecology of natural mothering.

We can't just drop out of our culture, but living within it doesn't mean that we have to adopt all of its practices. What I want to do in this chapter is show that the practice of mother- baby togetherness is preferable.

MOTHER AND BABY TOGETHERNESS

It is obvious that nature intended mother and baby to be one. In fact, a nursing mother who gives her total love and care to her baby will experience a relationship that she may never have with other persons. As one mother told me, "This is the first time I ever felt truly needed, that I was irreplaceable." This love relationship with its rewards is built in naturally—the mother's body is geared toward the giving by the continuous production of milk. Likewise, the production of milk provides her with a mothering hormone, prolactin, which is not available to the non-nursing mother. Nature has her own built-in laws for the child's development, and today her ways are being supported more and more by researchers in the field. For example, a chief ingredient for a healthy start in life is a continuous loving relationship with one mother figure. Nature has arranged this through the oneness of breastfeeding. Contrary to the popular opinion that you should avoid spoiling a baby, we are now being told that you can't give the baby too much love. Love him, enjoy him, fulfill his needs, and respond to his smiles, cries, and discomforts. Nature helps babies to receive this constant, individualized attention through the breastfeeding relationship.

46

It appears that some of our cultural theories concerning child care lack common sense and feelings. Mothers are sometimes told that they should let their babies cry, that it is good to frustrate their babies. The baby seems to be looked upon as a "thing" without feelings, almost lacking any human rights to be heard, understood, and loved. There are enough frustrations that occur naturally in everyday living without parents adding to them as a matter of policy.

Of course, all of this is done under the name of "not spoiling the baby." Spoiling a baby in this context refers to giving him attention of some kind when he cries or fusses. It is feared that he is just trying to get attention, which he doesn't really need, and is therefore being selfish. However, at his early age a baby's wants are simply the expression of basic human needs, both nutritional and emotional. A baby can't distinguish between legitimate needs and self-centered, unnecessary wants. When he fusses or cries, it is because he has a need that might very well be emotional rather than physical. Some writers have said that Mother Nature provided a built-in fussiness for babies so they will get some handling and comfort from their parents. Others have expressed concern about the "good" baby who is never picked up. The point is that love demands that parents take care of their baby's needs, and you don't spoil a baby by taking care of his needs in a loving way. Natural mothering provides lots of personal contact, and it is eminently well suited for taking care of a baby's needs.

The presence of a baby-sitter means the absence of the mother from her baby. This is not very easy in the natural mothering process because the baby will need her presence for food at least within a couple of hours if not sooner. Some mothers express their own milk, freeze it, and thus have it on hand in a bottle for the rare occasion when they just cannot be with their babies. The same holds true for the mother who simply cannot avoid employment outside her home. However, basically natural mothering means that a mother is with her baby—and baby-sitters interfere with this type of mothering and therefore with the breastfeeding-baby spacing ecology. Thus a mother who is interested in natural mothering and its related effect of child spacing will desire the oneness that nature intended between mother and child. She will soon discover that she does not desire to leave her baby; instead she wants her baby to be with her no matter where she goes.

The chief problem, of course, with following the natural mother-baby togetherness is not the enforced separation of the working mother. (By the way, in some of the European countries, employers provide nurseries so that mothers can be with their children occasionally during the day. A priest in Africa told us the working African mother has her baby right at her side. Such arrangements are rare in the United States.) No, the chief problem is basically a cultural thing that leads mothers to think that they need to be separated from their babies. There is a common expression of "being relieved of the baby." Many American parents make it a conscious goal to leave their children one or more times a week. It is considered necessary to do so in order to keep one's sanity or to maintain a happy marriage.

A friend of ours expressed dismay when she learned we always included the children in our trips. She informed me that getting away by yourselves as a couple once or twice a year was necessary for a happy marriage. This is what they did. Yet, sad to say, their marriage ended in divorce years later. Both John and I feel that the goal shouldn't be to get away from your children, especially when they are extremely young. Our two children were about one and three years old when she offered me this advice. We feel the goal should be to maintain your closeness as a couple without leaving your children.

I might also add that my parents included my sister and me on all trips and vacations; but my husband was often excluded from his parents' trips as a small boy, and this is one area where he wishes his parents had done it differently. So because of past experiences for both of us, leaving the children at home was not even a consideration. On the other hand, parents who desire some relaxation on their vacations will hire a sitter to go with them. Hiring a sitter in this situation keeps the family together. Other situations of hiring a sitter will be given later when the presence of a sitter is an advantage in keeping the family together for a certain occasion or activity.

It might also be asked if mothers require this relief from their babies. Dr. Thomas Lambo described the mothering customs of the African mother in an interview by James Breetveld for *Psychology Today*.[2] This psychiatrist says that the traditional African mother is inseparable from her child during its first fifteen months after birth. The mother meets her child's needs freely and even anticipates them before the child begins to whimper. Gradually, the child is given over to other members of the family who continue to give the child physical affection. Thus the child grows up in a secure environment of love and approval. The interviewer was interested in knowing if the African mother became irritated or annoyed with her child as a result of being with him continuously. Dr. Lambo said that, unlike women elsewhere in Western cultures, the African mother exhibited very warm and affectionate feelings toward her baby and that breastfeeding plays a part in the mothering relationship. With increased urbanization, Dr. Lambo is concerned that this mothering pattern might be changed in Africa. He stated that when women become involved in two roles, the traditional mother-infant relationship of inseparability undergoes a drastic change, and he is worried that this method of child care may be affected or lost to the African people. The report points out the fact that mothers can **enjoy** this oneness with their babies, that closeness and inseparability might play a big factor in this enjoyment, and that breastfeeding produces the environment for such closeness.

Mother-baby inseparability is a practice that produces happy mothers and happy babies. When asked why their baby is so good, some mothers tell people that it's because the baby goes everywhere with them. The mother's presence is what makes the baby so content! Mothers who practice ecological breastfeeding discover they want to be with their babies. Usually in our society mothers enjoy a break away from the baby. Not true for the mother who nurses her baby often. Being away from her baby is a very painful, unpleasant experience and she promises to avoid any future separation. The mother enjoys the togetherness and this special oneness.

One mother writes: "He comes with me everywhere. I enjoy taking him with me. I could not leave him as it would be like amputating a limb and leaving it behind."

Sometimes the pleasantness of mother-baby togetherness is contagious. One mother relates her story:

I nursed my first baby for four and one-half months (three months totally), but considered it a nursing failure. The baby did not gain well on breastfeeding alone as I used schedules and no lying down nursing. Our second was nursed frequently—about every two hours for the first year, slept with us, and went everywhere with us (including conventions, weddings, parties, meetings, restaurants, etc.). Our emotional bond is much different and I really enjoyed this baby. As a result of our example, at least three of our friends with previously bottle-fed, baby-sat babies are now following natural mothering and loving it. Having our happy, well-behaved baby with us all the time has been a joy and many people have remarked on this.

Another factor in this cultural advocacy of the separation of the parents from their baby is the mistaken idea that it is good for the baby to be exposed to a variety of people, the more the better, so that the baby will be social from the beginning. On the contrary, the baby needs its mother primarily, and, if an occasion does arise for a sitter, great pains should be taken to arrange to have a familiar person take the mother's place. Dr. John Bowlby, in his book on maternal deprivation, *Child Care and the Growth of Love,* [3] states that parents should not leave any child under three for a matter of days unless for grave reason. If the mother must leave, a close neighbor or relative should take care of the child; a stranger should not be chosen. Dr. Margaret Mead, writing on the subject of working mothers and their children,[4] warns mothers that frequent changes in baby-sitters may be harmful to the child. She stresses the fact that a small child needs care continuously from one mother or mother- substitute.

Maria Montessori, who dedicated her later life to the study and education of young children, appears to have been one hundred percent in favor of natural mothering and has some strong opinions concerning the early years in her book, *The Absorbent Mind.* She encourages only breast milk for the first six months and for the mother to take her time with weaning. In fact, she recommends nursing for a year and a half to three years for "prolonged lactation requires the mother to remain with her child." And she promotes the practice of inseparability by the mother during the early years.

For it is not at all paradoxical to say that, while adults suffer among the poor, children suffer among the rich. Apart from the complications of clothing, of social custom, of the crowds of friends and relatives that visit the baby, it happens that in the moneyed class the mother often entrusts her child to a wet nurse, or seeks other means of release, while the mother in poor circumstances follows the path of nature and keeps the child at her side. In a number of small ways we are led to see that things the adult world values can have reversed effects in the world of children. . .But let us think, for a moment, of the many peoples of the world who live at different cultural levels from our own. In the matter of child rearing, almost all of these seem to be more enlightened than ourselves—with all our Western ultramodern ideals. Nowhere else, in fact, do we find children treated in a fashion so opposed to their natural needs. In almost all countries, the baby accompanies his mother wherever she goes. Mother and child are inseparable. . .Mother and child are one. Except where civilization has broken down this custom, no mother ever entrusts her child to some else.[5]

Another author credits lactation as part of nature's way to keep mother and baby together. Selma Fraiberg, professor of Child Psychoanalysis at the University of Michigan Medical Center, wrote in her book, *Every Child's Birthright*:

The breast was "intended" to bind the baby and his mother for the first year or two of life. If we read the biological program correctly, the period of breastfeeding insured continuity of mothering as part of the program for the formation of human bonds. . .A baby who is stored like a package with neighbors and relatives while his mother works may come to know as many indifferent caretakers as a baby in the lowest-grade institution and, at the age of one or two years, can resemble in all significant ways the emotionally deprived babies of such an institution.[6]

To stress the importance of the mother's presence during the early years, some authors or speakers have made extremely impressive statements to show the effects of separation upon the child. Here are a few samples.

Edgar Draper, M.D., Chairman of Psychiatry Department, University of Mississippi Medical Center

If we assume that the sixth leading cause of death in the United States and the third leading cause of death in adolescence is not an inherited affliction, suicide must have its beginning in early life experiences. In the first eight months of life, an infant puts all its eggs into one basket, in the basket of the mother or surrogate mother, that I call 'thee one,' the one no one else will do for that infant. . .It's my contention that the first introduction to wish to be dead is when mother is not there and is not available.[7]

William and Wendy Dreskin, former day care providers

Full-time day care, particularly group care, is especially harmful for children under the age of three. For two years we watched day care children in our preschool/day care center respond to the stresses of eight to ten hours a day of separation from their parents with tears, anger, withdrawal, or profound sadness, and we found, to our dismay, that nothing in our own affection and caring for these children would erase this sense of loss and abandonment. We came to realize that the amount of separation— the number of hours a day spent away from the parents—is a critical factor.[8]

Theodore Hellbrugge, Director of Kindercentrum, Munich

The child's social development is always retarded if the child does not have a single main mother figure constantly about him, i.e., a person who has enough time and motherly love for the child. In this sentence, every word is equally important. **Single** does not mean two, three or four persons. **Constant** means always same person. **Motherly** means a person who shows all of the behavior toward the child which we designate as 'motherly.' **Main mother figure** means that secondary mother figures (father, brothers, sisters, grandparents) may support the main mother figure, but may not substitute for her. **Person** means that the respective adult has to support the child with his whole being and has to have time for the child.[9]

Hugh Riordan, Specialist in Human Communications; Director, The Olive W. Garvey Center for Improvement of Human Functioning, Wichita, KS

There are six reactions of children to separation when the mother is not around her child. The pattern may be 1) depression, 2) agitation or distress, 3) rejection, 4) apathy, 5) regression or 6) clinging. Why would a mother do that to her child?. . .When can a child withstand separation from the mother? Up to two years of age is a high anxiety time; from two to three years of age is a lesser anxiety time. This varies with the individual.[10]

Ronald Summit, M.D., UCLA psychiatrist

The risk of a child being molested "increases directly as the child is removed further from the care of its biological mother." [11]

These quotations plus others from twenty-two experts have been included in a brochure entitled "The First Three Years: The Importance of Mother/Child Togetherness" which is available from the Couple to Couple League.

It must also be noted that a mother who is with her baby can be extremely busy with other activities and ignore her baby's needs and responses. Maybe she is extremely preoccuppied with cooking, cleaning house, doing volunteer work, conversing on the phone, or watching television. One working mother learned to watch TV less because her baby would not nurse when the TV was on! It is one thing to take a few brief calls during the day; it is another to spend hours on the phone at the expense of little ones. I'm not criticizing the mother who has the occasional long phone call and nurses her baby in the process; I'm only pointing out that any excessive activity at home can mean neglecting one's duties as a mother. As one author appropriately said, "Busyness cancels out 'all-hereness'." In her book, *Your Child's Self-Esteem,* Dorothy Corkville Briggs further explains:

The opposite of love is not hate, as many believe, but rather **indifference**. Nothing communicates disinterest more clearly than distancing. A child cannot feel valued by parents who are forever absorbed in their own affairs. Remember: Distancing makes children feel unloved. No matter how we slice it, doses of genuine encounter pound home a vital message. Direct, personal involvement says, "It's important to me to be **with you**." On the receiving end, the child concludes, "I **must** matter because my folks take time to be involved with **my person**."[12]

CARRYING

When a mother brings baby with her, her baby is usually soothed and comforted by being carried close to her. I have come to believe that God meant for mothers to hold their babies a lot! Some experts say that babies have a high need to be near their mother and that this need is as important as their need for nutrition—and may be even more important. Inseparability facilitates frequent nursing and tends to prolong breastfeeding. Susan Dillman explained this association of carrying and frequent nursing well:

Species whose mothers leave their babies have milk that is high in protein and fat and they space their feedings from every two to fifteen hours. However, those mammals who stay with their young secrete milk which is low in protein and fat and they feed their babies almost continually. Human milk is low in fat and extremely low in protein, suggesting that the human infant is adapted to frequent feeding and extensive maternal contact. Because human babies are unable to follow their mothers around at birth and we don't spend months hibernating with them, scientists have identified the human pattern of infant care as that of carrying.[13]

Carrying also means a contented baby with crying being an unusual occurrence. In other countries where inseparability is practiced, crying is not observed. Yet, as Maria Montesorri brings out, "crying of children is a problem in Western countries," and parents often "discuss what to do to quiet the baby and how to keep him happy." She claims the child is mentally bored and "the only remedy is to release him from solitude and let him join in social life." Montessori explains in great length the many carrying devices women have used to have their baby on their body, and she also shows how the baby learns in a variety of ways when the mother shares her life with her child.[14]

Some mothers take this inseparability practice very seriously. A group of mothers in Arizona were followers of Dr. James Clark Moloney and his views on marsupial mothering. This former professor of psychiatry has written many articles on his views of

Mother and Baby as One   53

mother-baby "physical" togetherness. Having been exposed to his views, these mothers carried their babies on their person from birth on. Dr. Moloney felt that marsupial mothering should last for ten months or more, that babies thrive with an available, responsive, and loving mother, and that carrying or marsupial mothering was the best approach. His concern with the American mother was that many of them avoided such intimacy with their babies.

Some mothers have a small child that seems to need its mother all the time. I quote from the following letter to show that good things happen when a mother tries to meet those needs generously:

My fourth child had an unusually intense need for my physical presence. His need to have me available to meet his needs was very intense and long-lasting. He was so possessive of my attention that I really felt I ended up neglecting my other children (let us not even consider the housework!). I had to pour everything I had into meeting his needs.

This baby would not let me out of his sight. I tried to leave him with his father from time to time, but was unable to do so until he was 18 months of age. He either went with me or I didn't go. I was glad that I had three other more normal children because this baby was constantly on my body for the first 18 months of life. I used a Gerry carrier exclusively. I really needed the support my La Leche League group offered me, even though I knew I was doing the right thing by meeting all his needs. We left him with his grandmother about two times a year until he was two.

All the rest of society told me there was something wrong with me to produce such a dependent child, and there was something wrong with him for being that way. In brave moments I would just laugh and tell them that I expected great things from Joe, that the love you invest in children is returned to you and the world a thousandfold when they mature, and I had poured more love into Joe than any other child on earth.

Joe reached the independence of the average 18 month old when he turned three. We debated about sending him to school when he came of age. Obviously he was unable to stand the separation of school during the pre-school years. When he turned six, he reached another new level of independence and started the first grade the very next month very happily.

At the time of this writing, Joe is seven years old, and quite the most self-assured, independent, loving, thoughtful child you have ever seen. I know God has a plan for Joe. I'm glad I met his needs when he was a baby. I never could have done so without the support of *Breastfeeding and Natural Child Spacing*. I feel confident that if I had been unwilling or unable to meet his needs he would have been a very different person, equally as angry and evil as he now is happy and good. Thanks from all of us.

This story may offer encouragement to those mothers who have a similar high-need baby or for the mother who has several days where the baby seems to make excessive demands. A few mothers who felt their older baby was too clingy have mentioned later that much of the problem stemmed from their own attitude, that they did not accept their child's needs at an older age. Once their attitude changed, they soon discovered that their child's behavior changed for the better also.

Babies, even older babies, feel secure in mom's loving presence. The feeding embrace tells a little one that he is loved and very special, and the baby who has a mother who is readily available does not feel threatened by separation. This leads us to another advantage of inseparability: some of the breastfeeding problems are usually absent.

THE ABSENCE OF SOME PROBLEMS

Some mothers have written that their babies cry when they are put in their bed after being nursed to sleep. Some claim that their babies cry whenever they leave the room. Some notice that their babies cry upon awakening because they find that mother is not there. As one mother said about her baby: "When she realizes she's alone, she starts to cry." These situations are usually eliminated with mother-baby togetherness. The babies feel the closeness of mother's presence and do not fear that mother is trying to leave them. The baby is always with his mother. Very simply, where mother goes, the baby goes. And where mother is, the baby is. The baby who is always in close proximity to his mother is a very secure baby.

In our society this takes some adjustment in thinking. I know I went from "Where am I going and who will I leave the baby with?" to trying to leave only when the baby was asleep and returning when necessary for a nursing. The final change was taking the baby or toddler or small child with me everywhere, no matter what others thought.

The same philosophy can be applied at home. Running downstairs to do the laundry or upstairs to make a bed does not have to separate you from your child. You simply bring the small one with you. When the small one falls asleep (usually nursing to sleep), keep the child sleeping right in the area where you will be. This means that the child is not sleeping in his crib in a room separated from mom's activity or in a room secluded upstairs away from the household activity.

This idea of having the baby or little one sleeping near where the mother is may seem far-fetched, but in practice it is so convenient. I used a firm baby quilt placed on the floor in the corner or away from the flow of traffic. If it was hot, there was no need for covering the baby. If it was cold, I dressed them accordingly or covered them with appropriate covers. It was easy and convenient to lie down and nurse the child to sleep. After the child had fallen asleep I could easily get up without interfering with the child's sleep. When the child awoke or if the child fussed, I could respond immediately.

Mothers and fathers also have to realize that babies do not sleep all the time. Sometimes a baby is known to take only half-hour naps, sometimes an hour, and sometimes two hours. But soon they will probably be awake more during the daytime than asleep. A small infant who's awake can be carried around on his mother's person or he can be placed down on the floor on a firm pad or quilt near where mother is working. For brief work in the kitchen or laundry room, an infant can be placed temporarily in an infant seat and watch his mother work.

In the early or late evening, an infant or older baby can be nursed to sleep in the rocking chair and then placed near mom and dad on the floor. This is a convenient time for the couple to share their day with each other or their various thoughts or preoccupations. A couple who desire sexual relations that evening can leave the baby on the floor sleeping and then return later to bring the baby to bed with them.

Even a pre-schooler enjoys mother's presence while falling asleep at night. Dad may also be an acceptable substitute as the child grows in age. This time is a great way to end the day and to make the child feel good about himself if things did not go well that day. The time can be used for quiet reading, singing, praying or storytelling.

The practice of mother-baby togetherness also has an impact on child spacing. The following example helps to make this point. In a study conducted in the West African country of Rwanda, a culture in which there were no contraceptives or taboos against intercourse after birth, there were no differences in the birth intervals of bottle-feeding mothers in the city compared to those in the rural areas. On the other hand, among breastfeeding mothers, there were significant differences. Among the city mothers who were already developing patterns of separation from their babies, 75 percent conceived between 6 and 15 months postpartum. However, in the rural areas, mothers had their babies with them all the time, and 75 percent of the rural breastfeeding mothers conceived between 24 and 29 months postpartum. The researchers concluded that the only difference they could see between the two groups was the amount of physical contact the baby had with his mother.[15]

In summary, inseparability is the key to the natural mothering program. A mother has to be available to meet her baby's needs. It is also this closeness from which the other rules are easily followed. For example, frequent nursing—day and night—is a natural consequence of this togetherness. The result is prolonged postpartum infertility and happier mothers and babies too.

References

1. Burton White, *The First Three Years of Life* (Englewood Cliffs: Prentice-Hall, 1975) p. 264.

2. James Breetveld, "A Brief Conversation with Thomas Lambo," *Psychology Today*, February 1972, pp. 63-65.

3. John Bowlby, *Child Care and the Growth of Love* (Baltimore: Penguin Books, 1953).

4. Margaret Mead, "Working mothers and their children," *Catholic World*, November 1970, pp. 78-82.

5. Maria Montessori, *The Absorbent Mind* (New York: Dell, 1967) pp. 99, 104.

6. Selma Fraiberg, *Every Child's Birthright* (New York: Basic Books, 1977) pp. 28, 54.

7. Edgar Draper, "Potency of the Mother-Child Relationship" (La Leche League Int'l. Convention, 1981, tape 134).

8. William and Wendy Dreskin, *The Day Care Decision* (New York: M. Evans and Company, 1983) p. 18.

9. Theodore Hellbrugge, "Early Social Development and Proficiency in Later Life," *Child and Family*, 18(1979)120-130.

10. Hugh Riordan, "Parent-Reported Effects of Frequent Mother-Baby Separation," (La Leche League Int'l. Convention, 1983, tape 125).

11. Ronald Lindsey, "Sexual Abuse of Children Draws Experts' Increasing Concern Nationwide," *The New York Times*, April 4, 1984, p. A21.

12. Dorothy C. Briggs, *Your Child's Self-Esteem* (Garden City: Doubleday, 1975) p. 66.

13. Susan Dillman, "A Call to Arms," *Mothering*, Winter 1985, p. 92.

14. Montessori, *op. cit.*, p. 107.

15. Monique Bonte et al, "Influence of the Socio-economic Level on the Conception Rate During Lactation," *Int. Journal of Fertility* 19(1974)97-102.

7

Stepping Out With Baby

The mother of a new baby cannot simply drop out of society for three years. I doubt very much that the traditional African mother becomes a social recluse. The answer is as obvious as it is simple: mother takes her baby with her wherever she goes. However, such a simple solution seems to have two strikes against it. Many mothers feel culturally pressured not to bring babies with them to social gatherings; others wonder how they could take care of a nursing baby in public.

The problem of nursing in public is a matter of planning and techniques which will be explained shortly, but it sometimes takes conviction, courage, and character to stand up to the pressure of one's peers.

DISCREET NURSING

If this is your first nursing experience, you may feel uncomfortable nursing in front of others. I certainly did! As I think back, with my first I always had to leave to nurse in another room. There were times, however, when someone would say something positive about breastfeeding and encourage me to nurse in their presence. So I did, and I felt quite comfortable about it. As you nurse more and as your opinions and convictions about breastfeeding mature, you will find that you will be more and more comfortable with nursing outside the home.

The key to breastfeeding in the presence of people outside your immediate family is being discreet. Practice it at home, and you will soon find that even your husband may not know you are nursing when out! Actually, with proper clothing, a nursing baby gives the appearance of being a sleeping baby. A mother can lift her blouse or sweater up a little from the waist and the baby's body will cover the exposed area. If you're wearing a blouse, it is usually easier to unbutton one or two of the bottom buttons. A knit top is great since it stretches up where needed. And a blanket wrapped around the baby can be propped up in such a way as to provide a shield for the nursing area. Nursing can be so inconspicuous that no one has an inkling about what you are doing. There will be times when people will ask to see your nursing baby, thinking it's asleep. The baby may be asleep, but they will not realize when asking that it was at the breast.

For example, after the birth of our third baby, a friend dropped by to see my baby, and we sat down in the kitchen for a brief visit. Upon leaving, she asked to see the baby and was very surprised when I told her the baby was nursing. She was totally unaware of what I was doing since I had a very light blanket wrapped around the baby which provided some privacy. The baby was also covering anything below the nipple, and my clothes covered anything above. I have surprised myself at the number of places I have nursed my baby considering the fact that I once was so shy about nursing in front of others. You, too, will surprise yourself as you learn and gain confidence. The secret is to be discreet and thus others will be more comfortable with your nursing or they simply won't know!

I feel I would be very uncomfortable in the presence of a mother who nursed her baby with an obviously exposed breast or chest. There is no reason for such extreme exposure. Baby-formula advertising material often displays exposed nursing to discourage mothers from nursing. And, unfortunately, even many breastfeeding advocates show pictures of exposed nursing which can have a negative impact on a mother deciding whether to nurse her baby or not.

On the other hand, modest nursing sets an example that others may find attractive. One couple took their nursing baby to the childbirth classes they taught while leaving their older children at home. Some of their student-mothers decided to breastfeed their babies because of this example, saying breastfeeding looked so easy and could be done so modestly.

Certainly as a nursing mother you will want to consider the sensibilities of others. In a church service you may want to place your husband and other children between you and a complete stranger. Or sit on the outside aisle with your husband on the side where others would be sitting. If you visit a home where there are older children or teen-agers and you don't know the parents' attitudes about breastfeeding, it might be better to leave the room temporarily to nurse. There need be no explanations; just leave to use the bathroom with the baby.

Many nursing mothers feel that when female friends come over to visit they should be able to nurse in their own home as they normally do. Many have educated the neighborhood children as well about breastfeeding. When couples come to visit, again it's a matter of knowing how they feel about it. You may feel comfortable nursing in front of some couples when you entertain, and with others you will want to leave the room. I used to get angry that I had to leave my own living room to nurse the baby. It presented me with a double standard; if I were bottle-feeding, I could remain with my company.

One doesn't go against the cultural frown on public breastfeeding with ease or overnight. It takes time, and, as I've already indicated, there may be some situations—either out in public or even in your own home—in which you may want to nurse privately. Still, you will generally find that if you're quite casual, comfortable, and discreet about nursing in front of friends, they in turn will also feel comfortable.

Quite some time ago, I had established a friendship with a young girl, single and in her twenties, because of our professional interests. She soon found out that our two-year-old was still nursing and insisted I remain and nurse the baby during her visits to our home. Not until later did she tell me she was so impressed with my breastfeeding that she told everyone at the dental office where she was employed. The one thing she observed and liked the best about nursing was the ease in putting a little one to sleep. On some evenings when she would come over, John and I sat around discussing things with her while I nursed the baby to sleep. The fact that I didn't have to allow extra time or do any work to put our child to sleep amazed her. You may have similar surprises and discover you made a convert to breastfeeding by your discreet nursing among friends or acquaintances.

Other trends right now are making it even easier to buck the old taboos. Every time I see girls and women showing off their breasts in revealing tops, I gain more confidence in doing what I think is right with regard to nursing my baby. Why can these women draw approving glances for their detailed showing of the breast via skimpy, clingy, or see-through clothing while nursing mothers are frowned upon when they nurse their babies modestly in public without revealing anything? Our society has a distorted view of the breast, and it's probably our number-one sexual hang-up. Hopefully, this attitude toward the nursing mother will change as society becomes re-educated about the values of mothering and the important role that the breast has for the baby.

Once you have decided you're going to take your baby with you when you go out, the rest is fairly easy. First, when nursing outside the home, it helps to have the right clothing. Two-piece outfits, dresses with hidden zippers near the breast area, pants suits, ponchos, and ruanas (heavy coat-length wrap-arounds with front opening for baby which are ideal for cold climates) make nursing very easy. Never leave home, even for a short time, in an outfit that makes nursing difficult; your baby might surprise you and you'll find you're not prepared. Please see mini-catalog for "nursing clothing" patterns.

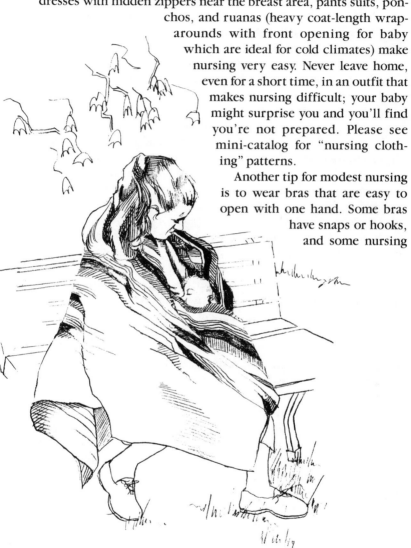

Another tip for modest nursing is to wear bras that are easy to open with one hand. Some bras have snaps or hooks, and some nursing mothers prefer bras with the "button" clip that can be easily opened with one hand. Since the most conspicuous part of nursing is getting ready or closing the flap, another idea is to wear a top you can't see through so one window flap can remain open. When our children were young, I often nursed on one side before we went out or before arriving, usually the right side. I could do more things while nursing on the left side, and for some reason I preferred this side when I was out.

In the early months leakage can be a bit of a problem. Nursing breasts sometimes get rather stimulated when you're out with baby, and in a short time milk can wet your bra and can make wet spots on your outer clothes. This can be a bit embarrassing sometimes, but there are a variety of solutions. The leaking can generally be stopped by applying pressure to the breast when you feel a let-down. This is obviously easier to do at home than in public, although you may fold your arms in a high position and apply pressure without anyone (except other nursing parents) knowing what you are doing. In another technique that goes unnoticed, I have at times applied pressure on one breast by placing my arm up toward the baby; the baby's body applies some pressure on the other breast. On some occasions a sports jacket or sweater may suffice to cover any leakage, while on other occasions you may want to use some pads inside your bra to absorb the leakage; homemade pads made from old cut-up diapers, hankies, kleenex, or other absorbent materials work well. During the early months when you go out, you can leave a pad for protection only on the breast not being used, and let your baby take care of the other.

Plastic wrap can also be used between the bra and your dress or blouse. Simply cut two pieces and tuck one in around the edges of each cup. However, the plastic cuts off all air circulation around the breast, and that can lead to sore nipples or can aggravate nipples that are already tender or sore. Because this technique can cause these problems, I almost hate to mention it; but some mothers with a heavy leakage may find this helpful, especially when wearing that favorite party dress that has to be dry cleaned. It need only be used for a very short time on that special rare occasion, and it should never be used during a breast or nipple problem.

YOUR SOCIAL LIFE

In our society child care is a controversial subject, and unfortunately many mothers who believe in what they are doing have been hurt by many unkind remarks. Some mothers have told me that they lost their best friends because of their differences with regard to child care. Though the situation is better now than in the fifties and sixties, the mother who takes her baby with her to various places and social gatherings still stands out as being different. The baby's presence says something about the mother's ideas about child care. It says rather clearly that she thinks that bringing her baby with her is anywhere from "good" to "the only way." Peer parents who have left their baby with a baby-sitter may be prone to make judgments, and self-justification may result in negative attitudes or judgments toward the mother-with-baby. Imagine the various currents and countercurrents when Couple A bring their baby to an evening at Couple B's house, only to find that Couple B have sent their children elsewhere to get them out of the house for the evening! John and I were in Couple A's shoes once.

As the baby gets older, it gets even harder. As one friend said, "You only accept certain invitations, those where you know the baby is welcome. But even when the baby is welcome, you know that the couples are wondering why you brought the baby, especially when he slept the whole time you were there. Yet, if the baby woke, I know how much he would need me."

You should be proud that you enjoy being with your baby and enjoy taking him places. You will find mothers complimenting you and saying, "What a good baby! Is he that good all the time?" As another friend said, "I hear these remarks so often when I go places with my baby that I begin to wonder if other babies are all bad." You will also hear favorable judgments from mothers who will say, "I could never take my babies [or small children] anywhere even if I wanted to." In other words, your mothering and breastfeeding helps to tell the world that maybe there is a better way to raise babies and that you don't have to be tied down while nursing! And you will learn to go places with your children.

When going out, sometimes it helps to plan where you will sit before you arrive. There may be some areas in a particular building or home where you would feel more comfortable nursing. Take a restaurant, for instance. Maybe the husband and wife want to celebrate their anniversary. I have known several couples like ourselves who have taken baby or the family along. This is quite easy, providing you pick a place that has reasonably quick service. Booths or out-of-the-way tables make it easier to nurse a young baby without being observed. A nice, dark atmosphere is not only romantic, but it might make for a more comfortable nursing situation. You may also want to select a place that has high chairs. The best advice to follow, of course, is to feed your baby if possible before arriving. If baby is sleepy and doesn't want to nurse, it may pay to wait until he nurses well and isn't tired before you take him out.

What do you do when you have to eat at a high class restaurant? One couple who turned down various business social functions and trips because their baby was not welcome simply had to attend a dinner in their honor. They wrestled with the problem and found an easy solution. They hired a babysitter—who came with them to hold and watch the baby in the lobby area next to the restaurant. They had a delightful meal and were at ease the entire time knowing mom was readily available if needed. The baby became the star attraction with the employees so the couple was also informed regularly that the baby was doing very well.

During the early months after childbirth it is helpful if your husband shops for groceries. To assist him, make easy shopping lists and let him do all the shopping in one store. When making the list, put the foods in the egg-milk-cheese section together, all the produce foods together, etc.; this will save him from making several trips back to the same part of the store. By going to the same market, he will become familiar with the best prices for certain products, and he will know where everything is for faster shopping.

If you have only a few grocery items to buy, you can place your baby in an infant seat and then secure the infant seat in a shopping cart. Make sure your baby is very secure in the infant seat and under your careful watch. Some of the infant seats today are rather large and the width may not fit as suggested. You can also shop at stores where the carts are extremely large and will easily contain baby and food. Many stores now have safety belts for toddlers in the seat section of the cart. When your baby is bigger and can sit up, a back carrier is very convenient to use while shopping. Common sense tells us that a hungry baby may soon turn fussy, so it's frequently a good idea to offer the breast in the car before taking him into a store.

Many mothers line up their baby's first baby-sitter when they go for their first postpartum checkup. Again this is not necessary. Some mothers may feel comfortable nursing in the waiting room, especially if it is uncrowded or has other nursing mothers. Others may want to make use of one of the several other rooms in the doctor's office. Once in the examination room, you can hand your baby to the attendant nurse during the exam or use the baby bed some doctors provide.

Wherever you go there will most likely be lounges, rest areas, dressing rooms, picnic areas, or isolated areas where nursing can be done easily if privacy is wished. If you have a car handy, this is also a convenient nursing spot. With proper clothing as suggested, you will find that once you gain confidence you may find yourself nursing along the sidewalk, on the school grass, at a picnic table, down mountain trails, or at the beach with a towel thrown over your shoulders. People will pass you by without taking notice.

The portability of breastfed babies makes them very adaptable toward social life, but certainly some forms are much easier than others. I would scarcely recommend taking a breastfed baby to a symphony concert—though I know music-minded couples who have done so without a problem, especially at concerts on university campuses. When it comes to family outings, it would be hard to find a better traveler. By age three months, one of our babies had been on two overnight camping trips in a tent, a trip to the zoo, a week's trip to visit relatives, and two trips to the doctors, and there were many quick trips to the beach, picnic parks, and the nearby wading pool. When traveling to other countries, there is no concern about the water supply, and couples claim that when flying great distances by plane, a breastfed baby requires very little fuss.

While babies are great on family outings, there are other occasions when a mother knows that her baby would be unwelcome, and it would seem best to try to avoid such situations. (Let me put in here a personal plug for not using your breastfeeding as an excuse to avoid gatherings and events that you really weren't interested in anyway. It may be an easy excuse, but it certainly doesn't do much to promote the idea of the real freedom of movement that the breastfeeding mother enjoys.) If you have to decline an invitation because you feel that the baby might be unwelcome, why not just ask if the baby is invited too? Then explain that you are limiting your social life for a while to those occasions when you can bring your baby.

HOSPITALIZATION

Nursing your baby away from home can occur during hospitalization of either mother or baby. But, it is usually easier when it's the baby who is hospitalized. Usually obstacles can be overcome and you can bring whatever you need to make your baby's stay more comfortable. One mother who found herself in this unavoidable situation said she headed to the hospital with "rattles, mobiles, toys, tape player and a determination to nurse a baby in traction" for two weeks and then through recovery from surgery. She found that adding a few props and pillows made it easier to lean over the crib to nurse; the hardest part she found was the long nursing in the evening because it was hard on her neck. Their two other children were cared for by her husband's family while her husband was working.

Today, many hospitals are willing to make arrangements in order to keep mother and baby together. A friend who had recently given birth was informed by her chiropractor after many treatments and tests that she would have to have back surgery to repair a disk. Her immediate concern was keeping her baby with her during recuperation. Her good fortune was this: 1) The hospital agreed to let the baby and father remain in her room during her entire stay. 2) Her parents took over the care of the other three children in the absence of both parents. As I have said once and I'll say again, obstacles in difficult situations can usually be overcome so mother and baby can stay together. And in both cases cited, the mother-baby closeness was maintained because of the husband's strong support, the support of family and friends, and the cooperation of the hospital. Compared to the hospitals of the sixties, today's hospitals are more open to promoting family-centered care in their maternity wards, and their staffs are more likely to have been educated concerning the importance of the mother-infant bond.

WORKING

Working—full or part-time—may bring breastfeeding into the office. More mothers are taking their nursing babies to their place of work with the support of working associates. Taking my last child to work two mornings a week was a breeze when he mostly nursed and slept and was rather immobile. Once he developed mobility, however, I was unable to work as the facilities were not geared for a crawling, curious infant.

Some businesses are such that an area can be set aside for quiet play and sleep near the mother's work area, and some mothers have had little difficulty in continuing their former working schedule.

For me it was a decision of working and ignoring my child at the office or taking work home and doing one or two hours a day at my convenience. Computers have enabled many more women to remain at home and produce work at their convenience. Some such mothers may own their own computer; in other cases, an employer may provide it. Other mothers who can't bring their work home find alternative sources of income. Many of these solutions are described in Mary Ann Cahill's *The Heart Has Its Own Reasons* and Coralee Kern's *Planning Your Own Home Business*. (See mini- catalogue at end of this book.)

Besides the Cahill and Kern books, another source of ideas for home businesses is found among homeschoolers, many of whom believe that home businesses are the ideal working conditions for Christians. Accordingly, this topic comes up occasionally in their magazines, newsletters, and workshops.

Some sorts of part-time work can provide a real Christian service as well as a bit of compensation. Nursing homes seem to be quite a growth industry, and our visits to a former neighbor indicate that these places can be very lonely; a high percentage of the residents almost never have a visitor. I've wondered if someone could develop a part-time business of running errands or carrying out special requests for these residents because a nursing home is one place where healthy children or a nursing baby would be welcome. And the same can be said of neighborhood shut-ins. Other examples of working nursing mothers are found in Chapter 15, The Mail Box.

VOLUNTEERING

Volunteer work is very conducive to breastfeeding in many different ways. One can teach breastfeeding or natural family planning classes which would entail as little as one night of teaching a month.

A variety of other services can be provided without leaving your small children home, and some of these experiences can be enriching for your children as well as for yourself. When our first two children were respectively three months old and two years old, I helped "pattern" a young girl, Debbie, one day a week. Our oldest child eventually became friends with Debbie, and about a year later Debbie was allowed to spend time at our house.

When our third daughter was three years old, the local Catholic grade school needed a teacher to cover topics on dating, marriage and family to two classes of seventh and eighth grade girls. No one else would do it, so I agreed to help. My two older children were in school during the time of the classes, so I took our three-year-old with me. Our Margie had a school bag of materials to play school with, and she loved being among the older girls. Needless to say, I covered topics such as childbirth, breastfeeding and mothering. Margie's only concern was that she did not want the girls to know she was still nursing! There were a few times where she got tired and fell asleep in my arms, but overall she enjoyed the two classes once a week as much as I did, and she especially liked eating lunch in the teachers' room.

When our family was young, I also visited a classroom occasionally to teach dental hygiene to small school children and brought my flip chart of "The Peter Rabbit Story." This visit was thirty minutes at the most and I always had one or two children with me.

Volunteer work should not be time consuming for a nursing mother but simply a brief outing that is enjoyable for you and your small children. Maybe you have an elderly lady on the block that would enjoy a visit once or twice a month. Maybe you have some talent you could share with a local school. One friend of mine volunteered to work one day a week at the school library if she could bring her preschooler. The school had never had this request before but consented, and the arrangement worked out nicely for both parties. The little girl enjoyed watching the older children use the library and was thrilled to have so many books at her disposal. One last point: be sure to tell your children how much you enjoyed having them with you and compliment them on their good behavior.

SAYING NO

The full-time nursing mother has to learn to say no. Because so many of her contemporaries are working outside the home, she can expect to be asked to volunteer for just about everything, and she has to become discriminating, to learn the fine art of saying no without offending people. You can politely decline some jobs because they would require too much time away from home or would be difficult to do with your baby or other children. Others you can decline because you already have prior commitments to other activities. Depending upon your personality, you will want to become involved in various activities to improve your community, however you define it. The only point I am making is that you will have to keep in mind the priorities of your baby and the rest of your family. Excess activity will mean excess fatigue, and excess fatigue can be a big factor in the early return of fertility. Learning to say no graciously is part of natural mothering.

CHILD ETIQUETTE

The behavior of your children away from home contributes much to the happiness or unhappiness of the trip or visit and also to the impression that "natural mothering" makes on others. Babies have real needs to be held and to be nursed; you don't have to worry about spoiling a baby by picking him up when he cries or fusses. Children under three have very real psychological needs for mother's presence; you don't need to worry about spoiling them by bringing them along. However, taking care of these basic

68

needs is a far cry from catering to their every desire.

For example, your child may have a favorite toy made out of metal or plastic—a great noisemaker when beaten against a wooden chair or floor. But you're taking him to church, so you substitute a soft toy instead. Speaking of taking your baby or very young child to church, attend a church service, if possible, that is more conducive to little ones. In addition to soft toys, consider bringing only those items which do not make noise, such as cloth books or books made of heavy cardboard coated pages, and have your child wear soft-soled shoes. Discourage your child from playing with the hymnals in the pew since flipping the pages can produce noise.

It might also be added that you can't expect a one- or two-year-old to sit still for twenty minutes. You expect little ones to be active. Much of the distraction comes from the parents themselves who expect their children to act like adults, and they are constantly disciplining their children. If your child is restless, you can carry them or hold them in your lap. Sometimes a little one enjoys a snack, and bringing along dry food (like small chunks of home-made granola) keeps the child preoccupied for part of the service. As a parent you can expect your child at times to be distracting to others during church. If a crying baby won't be quieted at the breast or a toddler won't settle down, simply leave the pew and go to the back of the church where you can hold and rock him a little as you stand there. Sometimes there's room at the back of church to walk a baby; pacing back and forth was comforting to our children. Also I found that it helped to stand near a colorful statue or a textured piece of artwork which caught the child's eyes and interest and the desire to feel and touch. Sometimes a brief walk outside helps. Certainly toddlers need to be taught that church is a quiet time, but parents should realize that happy, baby sounds are not distracting to others and that babies can't be taught to be quiet. You should be pleased that your baby is contented and enjoy his sounds—even though they do occur in church.

When visiting other people's homes, certain courtesies should be followed, and these courtesies are taught first in your own home. Teach your children not to climb or jump on furniture and that food and drink are to be taken only in the kitchen or at the dining room table. I had a La Leche League friend complain to me about another nursing friend who came over and allowed her toddler to walk all over her dining room table during mealtime! Children must be disciplined or shown how to behave. You don't allow them to carry a drink around the house nor do you allow them to eat in every room of the house. Even if you are renting a house or an apartment, teach them good habits in the beginning and your children will be more welcome in other homes. You will also have less work to do; no spills or crumbs to clean up in other areas of the house.

Another area of concern regards the child's movements. Some children are very close to mom and will be content to stay and play nearby their mother; others tend to roam. You must be responsible for your own children and know at all times where they are. Children can be taught to remain in the room with you during a visit and not to wander around the house. If they want to play outside or play elsewhere, they should ask. They can also learn not to ask for food when visiting, except water. Your job is to see that your child is not starved when you arrive. Children can also be taught to play cars and dolls on the floor instead of using good furniture, such as a piano. You can also watch that your child does not break any valuable items. Again, some small children can avoid touching nice items and others can't. Sometimes it's best to temporarily place the item out of reach of little hands and return it before you leave. Or you may ask to visit in the kitchen, family room or outside where breakables are not present. Again, try to plan ahead so the visit is enjoyable for you and your children instead of being a continuous source of frustration. After the visit find one area of good behavior by your child and praise him for it.

Occasionally, there may be a visit where everything seems to have gone wrong. If this happens, try to find something positive to say to your child if you can. If you can't compliment him, review the visit with him. Let your child know why you want him to act in a certain way, how his behavior affects you or others, and how much it means to you to have him come with you. Promise him a trip to the park if he improves on the next visit. Generally though, I think you'll find that with natural mothering, your outings go well.

PARENTAL RESPONSIBILITY

In all of this we have seen that breastfeeding and natural mothering do not confine a mother to the house or eliminate all social life. This is not to say that natural mothering does not make its special demands. Parents are mistaken when they try to act as if they weren't parents. The couples who continue to go away on weekends without the baby (or other children) or who keep up other life-styles that consistently separate them from the baby or other children for long periods of time seem to forget that parenthood carries with it a new dimension—greater responsibilities and greater joys. This change can be compared to the change from the single life to the married life. There are more responsibilities, more adjustments, and hopefully more joys to be shared. The husband or wife who acts as if he or she were still single or who does as he or she pleases without consideration for his or her spouse in marriage is immature. The parents who act without due consideration toward their new baby are likewise immature. On the other hand, the couple who choose breastfeeding and natural mothering are showing a certain sense of responsibility toward the baby by trying to do what is best for him even when it causes certain changes in their own lives.

For many couples, the occasional social restrictions of breastfeeding may be a long term blessing in disguise. Could it be that the abrupt severing of the physical relationship between mother and baby that is so common today is responsible in some way for the impaired relationship between many of our young people and their parents? We have all heard that the transition from the womb to life after birth is a shock to the infant. We have all heard of abandoned infants for whom the doctor's prescription was nothing more complicated or less demanding than lots and lots of loving care. The infant needs the loving presence of his mother, and this presence may sometimes entail her absence from a social event. If, however, the "presence demands" of breastfeeding are the occasion of providing a sounder psychological beginning for the infant, then what at first glance seems to be an infringement upon the parents' social life may very well turn out to be a distinct advantage for the child in terms of his later social life.

Breastfeeding may also help the parents to develop early the habit of thinking in terms of what is best for the family or for the child. In later years, for example, a parent may find that staying home is again what is best for his teenager. Parents today complain that they don't know where their children are; as a matter of fact, some children get concerned that they don't know where their parents are. Might ecological breastfeeding teach parents something of the value of staying home with their children and making the house a home by their presence?

In summary, the ecology of breastfeeding calls for that oneness of mother and baby that we have called natural mothering. Separations interfere with this. The mother has to be present to meet the various needs of her baby, and her continuous presence is the key to the natural mothering program and the maintenance of postpartum infertility. Thus, it is best for a mother to follow the practice of the typical African mother mentioned previously. For the first twelve to fifteen months the mother and baby should be practically inseparable. Baby goes where mother goes.

8

Weaning and the Return of Fertility

NATURAL WEANING

The time comes when your baby begins to wean himself from total nutritional dependence at his mother's breast to the stage where he is completely independent of her body as a food source. The mother who desires the most natural weaning of her baby and the benefits of natural child spacing has to realize that there are different methods of weaning and that one of these is quite conducive to natural child spacing.

In many quarters there is the practice of weaning a baby or toddler abruptly. One friend told me that she was advised to shorten the weaning process to one day. She was told by several acquaintances to refuse to nurse the child and let him cry it out. Presumably the baby would soon get tired of crying and take the bottle, which up to this time he had refused to take. Naturally, such a form of weaning would completely terminate any child-spacing effect that had been derived from breastfeeding and that might be continued for some time in a more gradual weaning process.

The natural means of weaning that can continue to maintain the child-spacing effect of breastfeeding is a very gradual process that is controlled largely by the baby himself. Although up to this point I have severely insisted that **total** breastfeeding is a very important factor in natural infertility, it is now necessary to point out that gradual weaning at the right time can extend breastfeeding's infertility considerably.

There are two key factors in what I call natural weaning. First,

72

mother has to wait until baby is naturally **ready** for solids; secondly, she has to wean her baby **gradually** off the breast at her child's pace. Early weaning—by which I mean not only hasty weaning but the early use of solids, bottles, or cups—may be gradual, but it is not what I call **natural** weaning. Nature apparently intended that the baby receive only milk from its mother in the first months of life. Any deviation from this natural plan, such as early weaning, usually brings with it a short history of breastfeeding. Short-term nursing among so many mothers today is why we hear the oft-repeated statement that women conceive while nursing. Early weaning means an early return of fertility after childbirth.

My own particular case points out the fact that gradual weaning alone is not sufficient to prolong the natural spacing effect **if** this gradual weaning occurs early when baby is still meant to have a milk diet from mother. With early weaning (use of the bottle, pacifier, and other practices not recommended in this book) I experienced menstruation three months after childbirth, even though I nursed for ten months and withheld solids until the sixth month. On the other hand, I found that by caring for a later baby naturally (total nursing until the baby wanted other foods and nursing often to meet the child's emotional needs), menstruation did not return until near the baby's first birthday.

When natural weaning occurs, some babies may wean themselves rather quickly; others will continue to nurse quite heavily for a long period of time even though they are eating many solid foods. **An older baby of increasing size, activity, and appetite may begin to take other food and still continue to nurse as much as before.** Frequent nursing may continue well into the second or third year of life. Since frequent nursing is the major factor in breastfeeding infertility, you can see how gradual, natural weaning can extend postpartum infertility.

If the baby is to set the pace, how can you tell when your baby is ready for his first taste of solid food? The answer is simple— your baby's actions will tell you when he is ready. A baby has an early desire to put everything into his mouth. There will come a time when the older baby, sitting on your lap at the table, will not be satisfied until he can have some of the food that he sees in front of him. Or he will start to feed himself with his fingers when he is ready. The same holds true for the cup. Someday he will want a cup and will make his new desires quite evident. In other words, you don't need to spoon-feed a child or offer a cup in an effort to introduce baby to his first solid food or liquids. Just wait and let your baby call the shots.

Normally, a baby begins to show an interest in solids during the middle of the first year. Some mothers say their babies wanted solids at five months; others are ready at seven months or a little later. Some mothers have found that their babies take only a little bit of food at first and don't really show a real interest in it until later. A mother may offer mashed banana or a mashed pea served on a baby spoon to her six-month-old only to find the baby pushing the food out of his mouth. The mother will then wait and maybe try again a week later. Although most mothers have been taught by society that it is "good" for baby to eat lots of food three times a day right from the start, nature as usual seems to set a slower pace.

Now that her baby is showing an interest in food, the nursing mother can still be flexible about her baby's needs. Just as there was no rigid feeding schedule while completely nursing, so there will be no rigid feeding schedule during the weaning phase of breastfeeding. She may offer him a little food once or twice a day; another day she may be surprised to find that her baby only nursed the entire day. Gradually, however, he will be at the table for most of the family meals.

The mother who is nursing has not had, of course, the mess of spoon-feeding a young infant, nor the problem of cleaning bibs or stained shirts. She will find now that feeding solids to an older baby is very easy. At the table the mother can mash the food with a fork, and certain foods, such as fresh fruit, can be scraped with a spoon. The mother will discover that her baby soon prefers his food in strips. These finger foods can be made from a variety of nutritious foods. She will not offer her baby sweet foods of the candy and cookie variety. She will avoid excess use of filler foods such as processed white bread and crackers. These foods may decrease her baby's desire to eat good foods, and they may be harmful to his teeth.

It should be remembered that the beginning of solid food does not mean an end to breastfeeding: **solids at first are only a supplement to breastfeeding and not a replacement**. Nursings will still be periodic and frequent if the baby desires them day or night. The baby may still want to nurse during the night or upon awakening in the morning. He may want his mother at the table during and again after a meal. The mother may be offering the breast for a mid-morning or mid-afternoon snack, and her baby will probably still want to be nursed to sleep. Breast milk will still continue to be an easy, quick nutritious food for the thirsty or hungry toddler. It will continue to be his liquid diet for many months. After he shows some interest in a cup, he will continue to nurse at the breast and may frequently insist on having a drink from his mother while flatly refusing any cup she offers him.

Babies will wean themselves off the breast naturally. A few babies finish weaning before their first birthdays, but this is early. Most babies wean before or after their second or third birthday. Others will nurse longer: three of my children nursed well past their third birthdays. Many people are upset to hear that a one-year-old is still nursing, but think nothing of a two- year-old with bottle in hand. Thus, when someone expresses surprise at a baby still breastfeeding past his second or third birthday, the nursing mother might politely ask her friend if she would be surprised if the baby had an occasional bottle or used a pacifier at that age. Toward the end of the weaning period it must be remembered that the child is not nursing every few hours but may be nursing only occasionally during the day—for example, before naps or during the night. The night feeding before bedtime is often the last feeding to be dropped.

There are a few other points I want to mention with respect to natural weaning. First, it would be wrong for a mother to withhold solids at her baby's expense or health. She should not consider prolonged 100 percent breastfeeding in order to prolong the absence of menstruation for a longer period when her baby really wants and needs solid food. Secondly, natural weaning does not mean that she will hold her baby back. A mother can't help but offer her baby encouragement over his progress. On the other hand, she will also realize that this slightly older child is still a baby in many ways and still needs to nurse. Just as she won't hold him back in order to prolong breastfeeding infertility, she also won't deprive him of his nursing in order to achieve another pregnancy. She accepts this "nursing" need of his approvingly and learns to enjoy this long-term relationship. (See Chapter 13 for further comments about this subject.)

Niles Newton concludes from her studies that what counts in a nursing relationship is the **type** of breastfeeding and the **type** of weaning.[1] Unsuccessful breastfeeding is that type of breastfeeding in which the mother calculates, regulates, and weighs the nursing experience. She constantly worries about her milk, when to give it, and how long to give it. The nursing is so limited that more breast problems develop. Weaning comes early as a result of all the bother. Successful breastfeeding is different. The mother feeds the baby as he desires. The milk is plentiful, there are no worries, and the mother enjoys the relationship with few breast problems. The unrestricting approach of this type of breastfeeding is more enjoyable, and thus the mother is in no hurry to end the nursing relationship. In addition, Newton questions whether the baby may be hurt by sudden weaning, as this means an abrupt ending to a close, intimate relationship with the mother. Thus, gradual weaning with its almost imperceptible changes may have psychological as well as physiological advantages. Mothers have found the practice of baby-led weaning very satisfying as indicated by the following examples.

Our two-year-old weaned himself recently. The first time he quit for a month: then he resumed for another month and now he has given it up again. I'm glad he did the deciding. It really makes me feel right inside. I know you know the joys of nursing a toddler, but this is the first time for me and it was so rewarding, so special. I do think God was very wise in his plan for babies and mothers. I'm wondering if perhaps the nursing experience doesn't help the weaning that must come when the young adult leaves home.

My youngest is now four years old and weaned about a week before his fourth birthday. He still has a little try once in a while but informs me I'm empty. I have enjoyed baby-led weaning so much and can see all the advantages so clearly. I only wish I'd been doing this with the first two, although they are reaping the benefits, too. I can't think of anything that's more enjoyable and rewarding than being a mother.

Nursing an older baby seemed to be a particular experience with me as Lennie didn't wean until she was three. Now my arms are so empty I find much joy in the children as they are growing and maturing, but there is just that special **something** about breastfeeding that we don't ever experience again.

RETURN OF MENSTRUATION

During the natural course of breastfeeding, a mother will experience the return of menstruation, for during the weaning process the baby will be taking less and less from the breast. The reduced frequency of nursings is probably the major factor in the return of menstruation and fertility even though baby may still be receiving a good quantity of milk. If the weaning process is a natural affair, the return of menstruation will usually occur while the mother is nursing her baby. If the weaning is abrupt, the return of menstruation normally occurs several weeks (two to eight) after the nursing has stopped. Any sort of weaning, then, brings with it the eventual return of menstruation.

The first sign of the future return of fertility is generally what we have been talking about, the return of menstruation. I say "future return" because ovulation usually does not occur before the first period following childbirth. Many nursing mothers have relied successfully on breastfeeding infertility during amenorrhea, and many mothers experience some infertile cycles after the return of menses.

The absence of menstruation provides a sense of security for the nursing mother who would like to avoid an immediate pregnancy following childbirth. This feeling of security can be lost if any bleeding or spotting occurs. Some mothers experience spotting or bleeding in the early months, but then increase the nursings to hold back menstruation once again. Spotting may also be a warning that menstruation or ovulation is just around the corner. Indeed, a few mothers have conceived after a spotting and without having had a regular menses.

Nursing mothers whose menstrual periods have not returned may be confused when they experience bleeding that is not menstrual in nature. The bleeding can be due to other factors. For example, one friend who had not expected her periods to return until the baby was about a year old experienced several days of bleeding much earlier. She then remembered that the bleeding occurred after a Pap test was taken. A check with her doctor confirmed this was normal; the bleeding stopped, and her periods did not return for months.

Another friend began cauterization treatments for cervical erosion. This "treatment" bleeding does not bring on a period, but it is confusing to the nursing mother who has not had any periods. The amount of bleeding varies considerably. For example, this mother bled seven days after the first treatment and twenty days after the second treatment. She was told that this "treatment" bleeding was all within the normal range. With such a lengthy flow, a mother can become concerned as to whether the bleeding is due to menses or the doctor's treatment.

A group of nursing mothers in our community some years ago discussed the fact that while they had all experienced an absence of periods due to breastfeeding, they were each surprised to have had a bleeding episode at about six weeks after childbirth. These mothers wondered what caused this bleeding since their menstrual cycles did not resume and they went on to experience amenorrhea as they had done with previous babies. Some of the women felt that the bleeding was caused by the resumption of coitus; others felt that maybe increased activity on their part was the cause. Most felt that maybe their bodies had not healed completely, and thus the bleeding occurred.

La Leche League shed new light on this in its 1981 revised manual, calling this six weeks bloody discharge not a true period but a "withdrawal bleeding" due to changing hormones. To reassure yourself that such a bleeding episode was just withdrawal bleeding and in no way associated with the return of fertility, I suggest making and charting the standard mucus and temperature observations of natural family planning for six weeks. If you have no further signs of fertility during those six weeks, you can discontinue charting until the signs of fertility appear.

The return of fertility does not mean an end to nursing. A mother can continue to nurse her baby or child while menstruating and even while pregnant. Many doctors become upset about the latter situation, but some mothers will continue to nurse in spite of their doctor's protest. It has been done for centuries and has not yet been proven harmful to the unborn infant if the mother has an adequate diet. Weaning, however, may occur naturally during a pregnancy. The circumstances may change during pregnancy, and either the mother or the baby will want to give up the nursing relationship. The mother may physically resent the nursing due to hormonal changes even though she had planned to nurse throughout the pregnancy. She may feel uncomfortable due to tender breasts or other physical changes, although some mothers will continue to nurse in spite of the discomfort because their child is not ready to wean. If a mother is uncomfortable with nursing, her child might accept brief feedings or reduced nursings if a good substitute such as back rubs is offered. The child may react to the changes in the milk during pregnancy: it tastes different, and he may lose interest.

Some mothers continue to satisfy the child's needs at the breast while pregnant and continue to nurse two children following childbirth. This is especially true in other cultures where breastfeeding is widely practiced. Several mothers have found that continued nursing is desirable from the standpoint that the older child does not resent the new baby. One mother wrote of her older nursing child:

Her complete acceptance of nursing as a fact of life for herself and for the baby is as delightful and useful a thing as amenorrhea—in that jealousy in its usual forms with the birth of a new baby has been minimal; any reaction has been more like intrigued attention at odd moments. That's been particularly refreshing to me since our first early-weaned child was a most unhappy soul for ages when faced with a similar situation. So not only did I enjoy a completely successful two-year spacing between children but also this added bonus of a happy displaced toddler.

A nursing mother when pregnant should consider the consequences of her actions. Is her child ready for reduced nursings? Do other activities with mother suffice in place of a nursing? Many nursing children, even the older ones, will not be ready to wean; and, if so, there is really no reason to quit. Actually, as we have seen from the above example, forced weaning may be most unpleasant after the birth of the newborn, whereas continued nursing may be advantageous under the circumstances. In addition, a child who has had his needs fully met by his mother and who knows his mother will continue to satisfy his needs and love him will be less inclined to be jealous; he has a secure relationship with his mother and the new baby does not pose any threat to his security. He is also more inclined to be concerned that the baby gets **his** needs met, too. There is nothing more touching than to see a young brother or sister be upset at the first cry of the new baby and insist that Mommy take care of baby right away.

I have also received a few letters from mothers who quit nursing during pregnancy because they felt they should. Later they were upset to hear that they could have continued the nursing. One such mother, who had a stillborn, regretted her weaning decision during early pregnancy. A mother likewise may wean and later experience a miscarriage. Breastfeeding will not affect a good pregnancy, but such situations do happen whether one is nursing or not, and thus these possibilities are worth considering when making a decision. On the other hand, these considerations should not lead a mother to feel forced to continue nursing during pregnancy. She should feel free to do what she sees as best, everything considered.

MENSTRUAL VARIATION AMONG MOTHERS

Why does one mother nurse her completely breastfed baby and have periods while another mother introduces juices early and still does not experience a menstrual period? Why does one mother whose baby uses a pacifier regularly not experience a period until her nursing baby is two years old while another mother follows all the rules for natural mothering and experiences a period when her child is five months old? Apparently the amount of mothering and stimulation required at the breast to hold back menstruation varies among mothers, some of whom require more stimulation than others.

There is also some evidence that the older a woman is and the more children she has had, the longer it will be before menstruation returns. However, this increase in amenorrhea is so small that one wonders if the experience built up over the years creates more confidence and, as a result, mothers nurse better and longer with each child. Better and longer lactation would tend to postpone menstruation a little longer. On the other hand, a few mothers have reported an earlier return of menstruation with advancing age. These mothers have nursed other babies, yet with their new baby they are disappointed when menstruation returns earlier than ever before. Some mothers who were following the guidelines in this book have told me this has happened to them.

Likewise, babies vary. Each baby has different sucking and weaning needs; some babies desire the breast more often than others. These factors are individual variations over which we have little control. However, they appear to be minor considerations for most mothers.

The most important considerations are those over which we have a great deal of control. Are we going to care for our babies at the breast naturally, or are we going to nurse but also offer breast substitutes? Are we going to follow the total mothering program? This is what will make the difference to the individual mother. Here is an example from a mother who used only breastfeeding to space the births of her children. Her first baby was nursed for eleven months (totally breastfed for five), had night feedings for eight months and used a pacifier frequently; menses returned at six months and conception occurred at twelve months postpartum. With the second baby the mother nursed for twenty-six months. Solids were offered at six months, but the baby did not take them until seven or eight months. This baby never had a pacifier and was given night feedings until twenty-six months of age. Menses returned at twenty-four months and conception occurred at twenty- five months postpartum. As we see here, a change in mothering practices can affect the duration of amenorrhea for an individual mother.

For many mothers the mechanism involved is a very delicate one. Any decrease in the nursing may cause a return of menses. Eliminating one guideline from this book may shorten or eliminate any natural spacing effect for a particular woman. These mothers require frequent nursing to hold back menstruation. Mothers who are giving total nutritional breastfeeding and who have experienced the return of fertility or menses are usually—but not always—not following the natural mothering program. One mother, for example, stated that she was totally breastfeeding and nursing her baby "all the time" when her periods returned. Upon further discussion it became clear that the mother fed the baby during the day only about once every four hours and the baby was already sleeping through the night.

Mothers who require lots of nursing stimulation will probably find that, once their periods return, they will continue to have periods regularly even though the baby may increase his nursing at the breast. However, there are other mothers who require very little stimulation to hold back menstruation. They can be down to only two nursings a day and still not experience a return of menses. In addition, once their periods do resume, a little bit of increased nursing at the breast may influence their cycles.

Increased nursings—for example, when the baby is sick—may delay ovulation in a cycle; thus the cycle would be longer than usual. Increased nursing may also inhibit or delay ovulation so that the mother does not experience menstruation again for a length of time. This type of suppression is more likely to occur during the first year after childbirth and less likely to occur after that.

This type of menstrual disturbance is less likely under the natural mothering program since the stimulation is gradually reduced and coincides with the baby's reduced sucking needs. The natural return of menstruation via natural mothering tends to provide more regularity for the nursing mother. Cultural nursing, with its use of artifacts as mother substitutes, usually results in a fairly early return of menstruation. For various reasons, including the variations in the young baby's sucking pattern, delayed and irregular periods appear to be more commonly associated with an early return of menstruation than with a later return.

Generally speaking, when can fertility be expected to return? Our research[2] shows that women who adopt the natural mothering program will **average** 14.5 months without periods following childbirth. This is only an average. Some, an exceptional few, will experience a return before six months postpartum. Others will go as long as 30 months without menses while nursing. Two women have reported their first postpartum menses at 42 months and one woman reported 43 months.

Some mothers who are well-informed about natural family planning and fertility awareness have found that even when periods return early, they charted many infertile cycles with continued frequent nursing. Thus for some mothers under the natural mothering program, fertility is delayed considerably even though menstruation is occurring regularly.

Those mothers who went for two years without a period are on the long side of the average in our study, but they are not abnormal; indeed, such extended lactation amenorrhea is common in certain cultures. One study among Eskimos showed that the mothers who nursed traditionally did not conceive until twenty to thirty months after childbirth, whereas the younger Eskimo mothers who adopted the American practices of supplements and bottle-feeding were conceiving within two to four months after childbirth.[3] When I wrote the first draft of this book, I felt that a lactation amenorrhea of twelve months was exceptionally long. Since that time I have met quite a few mothers who have experienced amenorrhea of longer duration, so that 24 to 30 months without a postpartum period sounds very normal.

THE RETURN OF FERTILITY

Fertility generally returns soon after a mother experiences the resumption of menstrual cycles; that's why the return of menstruation can be used as a general indication of the return of fertility. There are two exceptions: a nursing mother has a small chance of being fertile before her first menstruation, or she may have regular "fertile" cycles according to her charts and not be able to become pregnant until all breastfeeding has ceased.

As you can probably guess, there is an even greater infertility during the early months than later on. During the first three months of ecological breastfeeding and lactation amenorrhea, the probability of becoming pregnant is almost nil. During the next three months of amenorrhea and ecological breastfeeding, the chances of pregnancy are at the one percent level. The earliest return of fertility I've seen recorded by someone doing ecological breastfeeding was at four and one-half months, based on her mucus and temperature record and followed by her first period.

After six months postpartum, the chances of becoming pregnant with unrestricted intercourse before your first period are about six percent, assuming you continue with the unrestricted nursing of natural mothering. That figure is based on several studies. In 1897, Remfry[4] found a five percent pregnancy rate before the first period among Quebec breastfeeding mothers; in 1969, Bonte and van Balem[5] found a similar rate of 5.4 percent in Rwanda; in 1971, Prem[6] reported a rate of 6 percent among breastfeeding American mothers.

For mothers who do not desire another pregnancy at this time and are concerned about the risk of pregnancy prior to the return of menstruation, proper instruction in natural family planning can reduce that risk to close to one percent.[7] For mothers desiring immediate pregnancy, I would still encourage natural family planning charting because the sustained temperature elevation is the best indicator of your baby's age during pregnancy. This evidence can save you unnecessary tests and expense. First, you will know you are pregnant and thus will not need a pregnancy test. Secondly, knowing the baby's age can save money during the latter part of pregnancy should a problem develop. Oftentimes the number one concern in this latter situation is the age of the unborn baby. The temperature graph is the single most accurate method of estimating the date of conception and therefore gestational age, according to Dr. Konald Prem of the Department of Obstetrics and Gynecology of the University of Minnesota School of Medicine.[8] This information is helpful in estimating the date of childbirth for every baby; it's even more important in high risk pregnancies and when complications develop.

The general experience of those mothers with long periods of lactation amenorrhea is that normal fertility is not impaired once menstruation returns. The mother who experienced 43 months of lactation amenorrhea was most appreciative of the information found in the first edition of this book: "I would have never suppressed ovulation for three and one-half years," and "I could have wasted time and money in doctors' offices thinking I was abnormal." She found that once her cycles returned, they "have been quite regular and ovulation occurs each month." Many mothers also experience another pregnancy shortly after lactation amenorrhea ends, showing that fertility has not been impaired by the breastfeeding experience.

You may have heard that the saying, "a woman cannot get pregnant while nursing," is an old wives' tale or superstition. Too many doctors still express this view. I agree that a woman can get pregnant while nursing; however, this fact does not present the whole story. With the typical American pattern of restricted nursing, fertility returns quite quickly—frequently just as quickly as for the non-nursing mother. On the other hand, with proper knowledge and support, with the adoption of the natural mothering program, the average nursing mother will experience an extended period of infertility. If no form of birth regulation is used except natural breastfeeding, babies on the average will be born about two to three years apart.

References

1. Niles Newton, *Maternal Emotions* (New York: Hoeber, 1955) p. 49.
2. See Appendix II.
3. J. A. Hildes and O. Schaefer, "Health of Igloolik Eskimos and Changes with Urbanization" (Paper presented at the Circumpolar Health Symposium, Oulu, Finland, June 1971).
4. Leonard Remfry, "The Effects of Lactation on Menstruation and Pregnation," *Transactions of the Obstetrical Society of London*, 38(1897)22-27.
5. Monique Bonte and H. van Balem, "Prolonged Lactation and Family Spacing in Rwanda," *Journal of Biosocial Science*, 1:2 (April 1969)97-100.
6. Konald A. Prem, "Post-Partum Ovulation," (Unpublished paper presented at La Leche League International Convention, Chicago, July 1971.)
7. See Chapter 17.
8. Konald A. Prem, "Assessment of Gestational Age," *Minnesota Medicine*, September 1976, p. 623.

9

Getting Off to a Good Start

The most successful breastfeeding and natural mothering experiences are those that get off to a good start. This is not to say that mothers who have gotten off to a poor start cannot have rewarding mothering experiences, but it is obvious that it is more pleasant to have everything going for you from the beginning than to experience all sorts of problems.

There are various factors involved in getting off to a good start. Some have to do with the mental and physical preparation of the mother; others have to do with her doctor or midwife, her childbirth experience, and her advisers, whether freely chosen or self-appointed. Sometimes all of these favorably combine for a delightful experience; at other times a mother may have to be very determined and even courageous in order to arrange to have things working for her instead of against her.

THE MOTHER HERSELF

In conversations about the desirability of breastfeeding and its naturalness, the first question that usually arises is, "What about the mother who can't nurse?" I think that those who are physically unable to breastfeed are about as rare as those who are physically unable to swim. A mother who has had both breasts surgically removed would obviously be physically unable to nurse her baby, just as a person without arms or legs would be unable to swim. Also, a woman taking an oral contraceptive **should not** nurse because it may adversely affect the baby; furthermore, the "pill" tends to suppress lactation. However, the vast majority of those mothers who "can't nurse" are in the same category as those who "can't swim"--they have never learned how. Also if society looked down on the idea of girls swimming, we would have very few women swimmers. If society looks down on or at least does not encourage breastfeeding, we are going to have few women successfully breastfeeding.

There are many reasons given by mothers as to why they were unable to nurse. They had the desire, but they say: "I did not have enough milk," "My milk was too watery," "My nipples were too sore," "I have an inverted nipple," "I had an abscess," "My doctor told me to quit," and so forth. However, the real reason why these mothers did not nurse was probably their lack of information and the lack of proper advice and encouragement from someone who was familiar with this natural process.

Whether a mother nurses or not--or at least whether she gets off to a good start--may be influenced largely by the type of childbirth experience she has had or by the hospital policies that she had to abide by. For example, a mother may not have enough milk because she is severely restricted from nursing her baby at the hospital where she is staying. Maybe she and thus her baby were overmedicated during the birth experience so that the baby's sucking response was very poor. Maybe the hospital is giving her baby sugared water or formula in the nursery, and thus she is given a sleepy, full baby at feeding times. Perhaps the hospital has taught the baby to prefer the rubber nipple by offering bottles and pacifiers in the nursery. And, as the mother left the hospital, maybe she was handed a pack of free formula, a gift that might encourage her to use bottles when her milk supply is low instead of simply increasing the nursing. Unfortunately, the use of bottles will dry up her supply even more. Sad but true, some hospitals do not offer the nursing mother proper support. Instead they promote policies and practices that can be obstacles to a successful nursing program.

Breast problems such as abscesses, engorgement, or plugged ducts would be reduced in frequency if hospitals allowed mothers to nurse their babies as often and as much as the baby desired and if mothers were educated to desire this type of unrestricted nursing. Using the excuse that it will make more milk, some hospital nurses do not allow mothers to express themselves when their breasts are painfully full. Our concern, however, is not the production of more milk but the elimination of the engorgement or the excess milk to avoid the future development of abscesses or plugged ducts and, in addition, to offer the mother immediate relief by such expression. In 1968, in a Canadian hospital, I was greatly surprised to be bound tightly around the chest area immediately after the birth of our third child. The reason given was that this would offer support like a bra even for the nursing mother. Tightness around the breasts can lead to breast problems, so I removed this binding as soon as I left the delivery room. Certainly no mother could nurse her baby with such a contraption wrapped around her. This was one hospital I was glad I had made arrangements to leave two hours after delivery.

As for sore nipples, this problem can be partially reduced or eliminated by preparing or toughening the nipple area prior to childbirth. The nipples can be lightly rubbed with a plain wet washcloth at bathing time or a soft dry cloth or towel any time during the day.

I truly sympathize with those women who have experienced sore, cracked, or bleeding nipples. Having been too lazy to practice what I preach about pre-birth preparation, I have experienced the distinct discomfort and pain of nursing with sore nipples. It does help to know that this soreness will eventually go away and that there are things you can do to help yourself in this particular situation.

For one thing, you need not restrict nursing with sore nipples. The discomfort associated with sore nipples is usually experienced right at the beginning of the feeding. Once the milk starts to flow the pain subsides, and you will be able to nurse with little discomfort; thus you may let your baby nurse for a long time without removing him from the breast.

Secondly, proper treatment can heal the painful nipple area. I believe that it is important to keep the nipples **dry** -- free from wet nursing pads or wet bras and free from ointments. Most importantly, apply warm air from a portable hair dryer **frequently** especially after nursing and whenever it's convenient to do so. After trying the various recommendations for treatment of sore nipples, this "warm air" treatment is the only one that brought immediate healing and relief for me.

The best therapy for a plugged duct or a breast infection is to allow the baby to nurse as often and as long as possible on the affected breast in order to keep the breast empty. Hand expression is also an additional help. The worst thing you can do at this time is to leave the breast alone. Unfortunately and unnecessarily, some doctors recommend abrupt weaning or cessation of nursing on the infected breast. As soon as I felt an area on the breast was tender to the touch, I would let the baby nurse for a long time on the affected breast, and I would massage the area gently toward the nipple, and the tenderness would go away.

A few mothers have experienced a white "pimple" on the nipple

86

itself and have reported excruciating pain when nursing their babies. Some found that a severe, rough squeezing of the nipple area during a hot shower or hot bath helped to unclog the pore. One woman who frequently had this problem said she would squeeze and pull the nipple gently after a nursing to drain the last few drops; she compared this to emptying a spray can before putting it away. Another mother saw a dried milk crystal pop out when she pricked the spot and applied pressure. In these difficult situations, as with sore ducts and breast abscesses, the mothers found that frequent nursing helped to relieve the problem.

Women may complain about inverted nipples, but a truly inverted nipple is very uncommon. If a mother does have such a nipple, she can obtain a special shield that will draw the nipple out.

Other nursing mothers are led to believe that their breastfed baby should be on a four-hour schedule. When baby cries two hours later, they begin to think their milk isn't good enough for the baby who isn't satisfied with a four-hour schedule. What these mothers don't realize is that their milk is well suited to baby's digestive system and that it doesn't curd in the baby's stomach as formula milk does; therefore her breast milk digests so much faster than formula milk that her baby needs to feed more often than every four hours.

Several couples have told us that they had to quit nursing because their baby had diarrhea. They have been misinformed. A doctor friend who is well read on the breastfed baby says that a baby does not have to be taken off the breast for any type of diarrhea unless the baby is so sick that he needs transfusions and couldn't nurse anyway. It is, in fact, the other way around. One mother told me that when her baby had severe diarrhea, her doctor advised total breastfeeding. Later, when the crisis was past, he told her she would have lost the baby if she had not been nursing. What some mothers or their doctor understand to be diarrhea is sometimes just the soft liquid stool of a breastfed baby. This stool will remain a thick liquid up until the time the child begins solids. A baby was not meant to have a hard-formed stool. In addition, in the early days a baby may have several movements a day or a spotting with each feeding.

Later, couples begin to worry about the opposite; they fear the baby is constipated. As the baby gets older, he may at times have a bowel movement once every two or three days. There may be a few times when he will go even seven days without a bowel movement, but the stool is very soft when it arrives--and that is the important point. If a mother realizes that breast milk is utilized very efficiently by the baby's body and that little is eliminated as waste products, she can understand why it might take several days for her baby to build up enough of a supply of waste matter before there is adequate pressure for elimination.

There may also be a situation in which a doctor will tell the mother to quit nursing because of a drug or test that is required of the mother. It is extremely rare that a mother would have to quit nursing, and any such recommendation can be met with "But doctor, I don't want to quit." If he sees that nursing means so much to you, he is more likely to appreciate any possible alternative. So contact La Leche League, and most likely you will learn that nursing can be continued. For example, a friend who was hospitalized and taking three medications was told by her doctor to wean her older baby from the breast. She was very upset with this advice. I encouraged her to call a local doctor who happened to be on the La Leche League Medical Advisory Board. Acting on my advice, she learned that she could continue to take all three medications and continue the breastfeeding as well. Sometimes doctors are not well informed about a particular drug's effect on a nursing baby, and they recommend weaning for safety purposes without seriously looking into the matter or looking for an alternative solution.

Sometimes we are at fault because we fail to seek a second opinion. The mother who encouraged me to write this book weaned because she was scheduled to have a radioactive thyroid test; the doctors insisted on complete weaning before the test. Both she and her toddler were miserable during the two-week weaning period. She became painfully engorged; her little one was upset and frequently in tears. This mother had always been very active in her local La Leche League group, often acting as librarian. Through her local group, she found out later that weaning was not necessary and that nursing need only have been stopped for a short time. Why hadn't she thought to contact La Leche League right away? It never occurred to her! Often times we assume the experts or the specialized doctors are all knowledgeable, and we never think to question their decisions. When she learned she had weaned unnecessarily, this mother was even more upset because she had failed to look into the matter and regretted the complete and abrupt weaning decision.

Therefore, if any problem does develop for you or your baby which may influence the progress of breastfeeding, please contact your local La Leche League representative or call the number given on page one to make an informed decision and also to receive any support you would need for your particular breastfeeding situation.

Nursing problems are also more difficult to take care of if one is beset with lots of company. It's hard enough finding time to follow instructions given by a counseling mother without worrying about entertaining people. And any relative who stays with your family after childbirth should be pro-breastfeeding. One friend finally decided not to invite her mother out to visit when their third baby was born. With her first and second baby, her mother's presence interfered with her getting off to a good start. She would purposely go to her bedroom to nurse her child privately to avoid subtle criticisms by her mother, and her mother would come into her bedroom anyway. She could not avoid her mother and she claimed as a result she was never able to nurse properly. With her third child she was very happy at six months to have totally breastfed and considered it a pleasure to be in the situation where she wondered when her baby would start solids. She also had the pleasure of her mother's visit, but at a much later date after childbirth when breastfeeding was already well established.

Many parents are supportive, and for that we are most thankful. My mother bottle-fed my sister and me and admitted that she knew nothing about breastfeeding. I told her I didn't either until I read a certain book. She asked if she could read it, so I sent her the La Leche League manual, *The Womanly Art of Breastfeeding*. She came out to help me after the birth of our first two children and was extremely helpful and supportive. A common complaint among nursing mothers, however, is the fact that their mother or mother-in-law is so opposed to their nursing in the first place or especially to their nursing when the baby is older. In these situations, it is important for the mother to have the support of her husband and other nursing mother-friends. Her husband can also handle the responses for his wife. Sometimes joking is the only solution: "We know he'll start solids by kindergarten," or "I'm sure he'll be weaned by high school." By such ridiculous statements, hopefully the remarks will subside. But here is where the husband's support is invaluable, especially when the negative remarks and questioning are coming from his family.

My main intention, then, is to show that a mother who desires to breastfeed should be well informed so that she is likely to have a successful nursing experience. Her learning process should start during the months before childbirth. She should learn what she can do physically to prepare herself; and of equal importance, she and her husband should become psychologically prepared to meet the possible objections of well-meaning but misinformed or uninformed persons ranging from the doctor or hospital nurse to friends and relatives. On the subject of breastfeeding, all too many people who have never read a book or who have never nursed feel qualified to pass on advice. On the other hand, the La Leche League has a professional board of medical advisers, plus the experience of thousands of women. Many mothers are most appreciative for the help and information they received from this organization. Having the right answer and support at the right time can mean success instead of failure.

Young mothers today may also lack confidence in themselves. Some have called me after they are home from the hospital to express a general feeling that everything is wrong. In the beginning of the conversation I begin to wonder if I can be of any help at all, but then soon realize that there really is no problem. Toward the end of the conversation I begin to see a completely different picture of a mother who is doing a fine job and who has a good baby, and I tell her so. These mothers only require a little more time to develop the self-confidence they need. It takes a little while for a first-time nursing mother to forget about rules and time schedules, and until this happens the mother does not really relax and enjoy her baby. At any rate, all that most of these mothers need is a lot of praise and someone telling them that they are doing what is best for their baby.

For those few mothers who may not be able to nurse their child, much of the motherly advice in this book can still be followed. The philosophy of giving of yourself, being close and in touch with your child, taking him with you as much as possible, holding him for the bottle-feedings and enjoying and loving him are the best "gifts" you can give your small child. A bottle-feeding mother can be a good mother, and there is no guarantee that breastfeeding always produces a good mother. However, if everything else is equal, it's just easier to practice good mothering the natural way of breastfeeding.

THE DOCTOR

What is the role of the physician in breastfeeding? Certainly, his influence is considerable with most mothers. He is therefore in an excellent position to foster the practice of breastfeeding and natural mothering. He can explain to the mother how her milk is the best food for the baby; he can tell her all the health advantages to both the baby and herself through breastfeeding; he can tell her about natural mothering and the natural infertility of ecological breastfeeding. He can assure her that she will be able to do a good job: he might recommend attending La Leche League meetings during pregnancy. He can tell her how much money she will save by not using bottles, formulas, and baby foods, and he might even tell her that it would be worthwhile for her to spend some of her savings to buy this book!

If you live in an area served by several doctors, then you have the opportunity of selecting a doctor to better serve you. You can ask other successful nursing mothers about their family doctors or pediatricians. Other good referral sources are childbirth instructors, midwives, or La Leche League leaders. You will want to know which doctors encourage total breastfeeding and which ones will go along with long-term nursing.

If you already have a relationship of long standing with a particular doctor, you may want to stay with him even if he's not as informed and supportive as you might wish. If he knows you, he may be quite interested in your new ideas and quite receptive to your complete breastfeeding. One mother expressed concern as to what her doctor's reaction might be to complete breastfeeding since he had put her previous babies on solids within several weeks after birth. She later told me that he went along with her although he mentioned solids at each visit, but he jokingly told her, "You know more about it than I." Such a doctor may be more open to a mother he already has a good relationship with than he might be to a total stranger.

On the other hand, there are still a few physicians whose habit of recommending early solids and liquid supplements is very strong. If your doctor should be one of those who recommends solids or juice soon after birth, you might ask him why breastmilk isn't sufficient. Many doctors will go along with the mother if she expresses her feelings on the matter in a gentle, sincere manner. However, if you think your physician may become authoritarian if you don't go along with his ideas, you may find it helpful to have your husband present for moral support. If your doctor should be particularly insistent, you may choose several alternatives. You might ask him for the research that backs up his apparent contention that normal mother's milk alone in the early months isn't sufficient. Since there isn't any such research, you may be putting him in a very defensive position. Perhaps a more diplomatic way might be to say that you understand that there has been considerable research supporting the idea that total breastfeeding for the first six months is the best nutrition and that anemia is rare in the breastfed baby. Some mothers choose to handle it one month at a time by saying, "The baby is doing so well, doctor--wouldn't it be possible to continue this way a while longer?" Others who have the strength of their convictions just ignore the doctor's advice, relying on his compliments about the health of the baby at the regular visits as confirmation of their baby care through total breastfeeding. Still others will simply change doctors.

In selecting a doctor for childbirth, you will want to be extremely careful in your selection. Again, you will do well to ask questions of local childbirth instructors and La Leche League leaders. Secondly, don't accept vague generalizations when seeking information. Get specifics. For example, I was told that a childbirth instructor discouraged a mother from going to my doctor because he was "radical." No specifics were given as to why he was radical. So you can ask again, "Why is he radical?" Keep asking for specifics until you are satisfied. It also must be remembered that we are all different and even the best doctors have bad days; therefore, there is always going to be someone who is unhappy with a doctor you think is wonderful.

Another serious consideration today are the doctor's values. Many mothers now are selecting only those doctors who are pro-life and also those hospitals that do not perform abortions. It is also a well-known fact that even some Catholic hospitals perform sterilizations. In talking to young mothers, I understand that there is a great deal of pressure by some doctors, even those associated with Catholic hospitals, to have a tubal right after giving birth. The C-section birth is so common today that such doctors like to get in the additional operation and money at their convenience. Some doctors not only apply pressure near childbirth time but are now asking the "tubal" question early in pregnancy. On the other hand, you would think that obstetricians who are pro-life and pro-natural family planning would also abide by nature as much as possible during childbirth. Unfortunately, that's not always the case, and some may have a high C-section rate, use forceps routinely, etc. All of the various options have to be considered according to your priorities.

One of the best referral sources is NAPSAC International (National Association of Parents and Professionals for Safe Alternatives in Childbirth), a non-profit, educational service organization which is also pro-life. If you are interested in finding a midwife, nature-oriented doctor, birth center, home birth program or family-centered hospital, you will want to purchase the *NAPSAC Directory of Alternative Birth Services and Consumer Guide.*[1] It lists thousands of practitioners and educators by state and community; addresses and phone numbers are provided. Best of all, the first thirty-eight pages comprise a consumer guide which lists questions a couple should ask the doctor, midwife or hospital in an effort to determine whether that particular service or practitioner is competent and desirable.

THE CHILDBIRTH EXPERIENCE

Another way in which a doctor can be either most helpful or most uncooperative for the prospective nursing mother is in the process of childbirth itself. Under healthy, normal, natural conditions, a new baby should be nursing within a few minutes after childbirth. This is just as much for the mother's benefit as for his because his sucking helps her uterus to contract and thus shut off the maternal blood vessels that formerly took care of him. In brief, that means that your baby's sucking helps to prevent you from hemorrhaging, and your baby receives more iron as the placenta is slowly detaching from the uterine wall. Your baby's continued suckling in the next 24 to 48 hours gives him the benefits of a fluid called **colostrum** while it continues to put your uterus back into shape. Colostrum is the name given to the first milk secreted by the breast; it is much richer and creamier than the milk that soon follows and which, by the way, may look thinner than the milk you would buy in the store, an appearance that does not, however, discredit its value.

I cannot emphasize too strongly that a mother should allow her baby to breastfeed without restriction during the first twenty- four hours after delivery. If you want a successful nursing experience, start early. Don't be surprised if your baby doesn't nurse a minute or so after his birth. He will do better a few minutes later. At a minimum, your baby should be allowed to nurse within the first half-hour after birth and at least every three hours thereafter. Preferably the baby will remain in bed with you and nurse on and off to his heart's content. This is the advantage of being home since remaining close to your baby is easier.

In order for mother and baby to have this good start at nursing, they both should be physically able right after the birth. Thus I recommend a prepared, natural, and--if possible--completely unmedicated childbirth as the best start for a successful breast-feeding experience. A mother who is unconscious from anesthesia cannot breastfeed. Just as importantly, her baby may have been adversely affected by the anesthetic used on her. Respiratory distress in the newborn has long been known to be caused by obstetrical medication. Furthermore, "sedatives containing barbiturates administered to the mother during labor have been shown to adversely affect the infant's sucking reflexes for 4 to 5 days after birth."[2] Thus the mother should begin nursing right after birth with an alert, undrugged baby. That in turn means she has to have a physician who will, first of all, allow her to nurse after childbirth and who will also assist the delivery in such a way as to leave both her and the baby **able** to nurse. The next thing she normally needs from her physician is the **absence** of a shot to contract her uterus: baby's sucking takes care of that. Then she needs the **absence** of any kind of a shot to dry up her milk supply. None of this seems to be asking very much, but a mother may have to shop around before finding a doctor who will be agreeable. Or better yet she can seek the services of a midwife or homebirth doctor and avoid the hassles of a hospital delivery by choosing to give birth at home. Or she may have the option to use an alternative birthing center.

THE HOSPITAL

Hospitals provide the first environment for the vast majority of newborn babies and their mothers. The official policies of the institutions and the personal attitudes of the nurses can have a significant influence on the success of breastfeeding. Each of these sources can be helpful; yet it is the unfortunate fact that too frequently they are either of no help or are actively detrimental.

When I wrote the first edition in 1968, I didn't have many nice things to say about hospitals with regard to childbirth procedures or infant care. However, there has been a widespread trend to accommodate those couples who desire the natural approach in childbirth and breastfeeding. Still, my primary advice in 1968 remains valid: 1) choose the hospital that will offer you the most support, and 2) leave the hospital as soon as possible. If you had a medicated delivery, then wait until the effects of the drug have worn off and until you are feeling well. 3) Consider a home birth if that is an option in your area.

Whenever I tell people that I came home within six hours after the birth of our two babies born in 1968 and 1972, I receive looks of utter disbelief. In both cases in two different cities, I was apparently the first such patient for each doctor, but there was no problem. My husband and I had simply talked about this with the doctor during my prenatal visits and requested that I be allowed to go home a few hours after delivery if everything was medically satisfactory with both me and the baby. By showing my willingness to stay in the hospital if either my baby or I really needed its special care facilities, I put the doctor at ease; on the other hand, he would have to have some medically valid reason (for example, something wrong with either me or the baby) in order to keep us in the hospital. In each case, both the baby and I were medically in good shape, and we went home.

Such ideas didn't originate with me. Rather, I was influenced first of all by the writings of doctors who have related their experiences with such practices and secondly by mothers who chose to have home deliveries in order to avoid any hospital interference. By going home early, you do get more rest than you would in the hospital with its many interruptions from the hospital personnel, baby photographers, etc. In addition, when you sign out, be sure to tell the hospital not to give your name out if you want to avoid the many sales calls that occur after the birth of a baby. At home your baby is tucked into bed with you; he is likewise not being exposed to possible infection in the hospital nursery. Your husband should be glad that he doesn't have to plan any more trips to the hospital, and in some cases he doesn't have to arrange for babysitters while doing so. Any children you have will appreciate your being home and being able to enjoy "their" baby too.

Rooming-in presents the best alternative to going home within a few hours after birth. If such a program isn't available, a policy of bringing the baby to the mother or of allowing the mother to go to the baby to nurse in a special room off the nursery for all feedings is the next best thing. The breastfeeding baby will benefit from the rich colostrum and will have a nice soft nipple for easy learning until your milk comes in. His frequent nursing will help to relieve or minimize the engorgement that frequently results from an unnatural separation of mother and baby.

The hospital environment can play a crucial role in helping or hindering the nursing couple. As I have stressed throughout this book, the only schedule in natural breastfeeding is the baby's. Thus the hospital atmosphere conducive to breastfeeding will be the one that allows the mother and baby to remain together as much as possible.

Many hospitals are now asking patients for an evaluation of their services. Whether it is asked for or not, it would be helpful to write the hospital complimenting it on its good points but also expressing your interests in other services you hope they will have or policies you hope they will change in the near future. It is amazing how fast hospital policy can change in a short period of time; the hospitals have become generally very receptive to what the consumer wants, and with the declining birth-rate and inflationary costs, they have additional reasons to listen. If the hospital charges you for medications and services not used because you left the hospital shortly after delivery, make a phone call to the billing department even if it is covered by insurance.

Perhaps a few reflections on my own experiences can illustrate some of the things a mother may encounter by way of doctors and hospitals. Because our family has been one of those mobile ones you read about in the statistics, I have had a variety of experiences, including a different doctor for each of our first four children. Our first doctor discouraged the natural-spacing effects of breastfeeding, and he was highly critical of the available natural childbirth classes in the area. I went to the classes anyway and was extremely grateful for having done so. It was also at these classes that I was introduced to La Leche League, an organization that made a good impact on our family.

Our second doctor encouraged the total breastfeeding rule for family planning purposes, but he discouraged rooming-in and husbands in the delivery room. He did leave orders that our baby was not to receive supplements in the nursery room, and these orders were apparently followed. However, I still wanted to try the other system so I switched to rooming-in before going home and found it a great improvement.

With our third baby on the way, we were now Canadian residents and had been informed that women stay in the hospital for three to five days after the "delivery day" providing everything goes well. If a woman had a C-section or had other complications, she stayed at the hospital for a week. This was completely different from the California hospitals where discharge occurred about 48 hours after childbirth in the mid-sixties. Now I wanted to leave the hospital two hours after childbirth and a personal doctor friend agreed to go along with my desires.

However, I was led to ask him specific questions when I learned at the childbirth classes that certain procedures were routinely done at birth. As a result I found out that our doctor would catherize me before and after birth and administer a shot as well to contract the uterus even with immediate breastfeeding. Fortunately, I had had prior experience with two cooperative obstetricians before encountering this anesthesiologist-turned-general practitioner, and neither of the first two had made such suggestions. This third doctor, up to the time of this, my eighth month of pregnancy, had been very cooperative, but now he turned tough, perhaps thinking that he could do as he pleased with me at this stage of the game. With my husband's support I terminated the relationship at that point and found another doctor who was cooperative.

With our fourth baby, my husband was allowed to observe the birth for the first time. With this baby, alertness paid off. I was taking care of the baby on the delivery table when out of the corner of my eye I saw the nurse approach me from behind with a long needle in her hand. I immediately asked her what it was for, and she said it was to contract the uterus. I told her I never had it with my other three babies, and the doctor then told her I didn't need it. Obstetrical medication is so routine that even when you have the best of natural childbirth doctors, you still have to be alert about the hospital personnel.

Our fifth child was born at home with the entire family present, and John and I were delighted that we did not have to go to the hospital. We had also learned through studies and books that the safest place to have a baby is at home.

YOUR DOCTOR'S C-SECTION RATE

An expectant couple would do well to ask any doctor who might be present at the birth of their child what his C-section rate is. According to the Public Citizen Health Research Group which is affiliated with the Ralph Nader organization, 455,000 C-sections were done unnecessarily in 1986. They also claim that "the national C-section rate has more than quadrupled in the last 16 years."[3] Most of the variations in the C-section rate, the group found, were due to the various policies of physicians and hospitals.

Hopefully this information will continue to remain in the news media so that consumers (those who will be having babies) will become better informed and will be in a better position to protect themselves. By the year 2000, it is estimated that almost half of older mothers will have a C-section birth in spite of the fact that this surgical birth costs $1,500 more and requires more recovery days in the hospital and longer recuperation. According to these projections, in the year 2000 40% of women aged 25-29 will undergo a C-section when giving birth to their children. For a mother who is 30-34 years old, the chances are 45% that she will have a C-section: for women who are 35 years or older, the C-section rate in the year 2000 is estimated at 49%.[4] Also many mothers today usually have a repeat Cesarean, despite studies which show that "vaginal delivery after a previous Cesarean delivery is just as safe for the baby" and "two to four times safer for the mother."[5]

The increased rate of C-sections should be a concern to all of us. I personally get upset everytime I think about it. I have learned that by many physicians' standards today I would have had my first baby by C-section. And like many women, if I had my first baby today, I am sure I would have believed that the C-section was necessary.

VERTICAL BIRTHING

It is my conviction that the upright or vertical position during labor and delivery reduces the C-section rate. It certainly facilitates labor and birthing. Other benefits include less tearing, improved fetal blood supply and less need for intervention.[6] Regarding less tearing and episiotomies, those who have had both the episiotomy and then later experienced a slight tear without the episiotomy find that it is easier on the body and less painful to experience a slight tear with its appropriate repair than to undergo another episiotomy.

The vertical position is more comfortable and easier for the mother-to-be as she has gravity working for her. With labor usually shortened, she has more energy as well.

Connie Livingston points out that "a position such as squatting can ease the process by increasing the opening of your pelvic bones as much as .5-2.5 centimeters."[7] By upright position, I am not referring to the flat-on-your-back position with head or shoulders elevated slightly and legs up in the air duing delivery. I mean that your body torso is in a vertical position for labor and delivery; such vertical positions are sitting, standing, kneeling and squatting.

OTHER ADVISERS

In addition to medical doctors, a mother may seek and receive advice from other persons. She may be seeking information about family planning, about breastfeeding for its own sake, or about breastfeeding as a means of family planning. Her advisers may range from her clergyman to the mother-in-law of the gal three doors down the street. In addition to these personal forms of advice, a mother or prospective mother may seek information from various courses offered in the community. Schools, colleges, and churches offer courses on marriage and family life, and frequently they have the opportunity to touch upon baby care, parenthood, and family planning.

Prenatal classes are offered in many communities, and the teacher here can greatly influence her students. One class I attended during my first pregnancy encouraged mothers to nurse their babies, and everyone wanted to nurse except one. However, in a similar class in a different city four years later, breastfeeding was hardly mentioned. The instructor, a nurse, spent some time passing out nipples and bottles--so the mothers would know how to put them together!--and toward the end of the classes she handed out family planning literature, remarking: "If you want to plan a family, don't breastfeed." In this class, only two mothers showed any interest in nursing their babies. Since the instructor never gave her students one positive reason why they should breastfeed, very few had the desire.

Clergymen are sometimes asked for guidance about family planning. It would seem that at least they should not discourage the natural plan of baby care and of baby spacing. More affirmatively, they should know enough about the natural plan to be able to describe what is involved and encourage couples to attend the natural family planning classes taught by the Couple to Couple League where proper information with regard to breastfeeding will be provided.

Various marriage and family courses provide an excellent opportunity to educate groups of people, women and men, who are open and receptive to the ideas of natural breastfeeding. It is important in this regard that proper attitudes and information about breastfeeding should not be limited to women. Men, too, should learn all the advantages of breastfeeding since the understanding and encouragement of a husband can be a great help to the nursing mother.

In our society, if the case for breastfeeding and natural mothering were made with the same emphasis given to bottles, baby foods, the pill and other forms of contraceptives, I feel that the desires of many mothers to breastfeed would remain alive. Many couples do not consider breastfeeding because they were never presented with any reasons for doing so. A good educational program could change that picture.

In short, nurses and doctors, clergymen, relatives and teachers, hospitals, schools and churches all play a part in the decision of a mother to nurse her baby and secondly to breastfeed in such a manner that it becomes an excellent means of spacing babies and, most importantly, of caring for babies. These people and institutions can either help greatly by inducing positive attitudes and imparting factual information about this natural process, or they can do the reverse.

Where does a couple go to find support and information with regard to breastfeeding and the related areas of childbirth and the natural spacing of babies? Couples who are interested in getting off to a good start can find support from three non-profit organizations, each of which has its own specialty but overlaps into related areas.

The Couple to Couple League International (CCL)

Natural family planning (NFP) is the specialty of CCL; however, since breastfeeding is the world's oldest form of natural family planning, and since childbirth practices definitely affect the breastfeeding experience, CCL has long been interested in promoting the best in each of these areas. Its NFP classes are taught by professionally trained volunteer user-couples; a home study course is available for those who cannot attend classes. My husband and I founded this organization, and we wrote its learner's manual, *The Art of Natural Family Planning*. In both the CCL classes and in its manual, we promote ecological breastfeeding and teach how to detect the return of fertility after childbirth, whether early or late.

La Leche League International

This organization is dedicated to helping mothers learn "the womanly art of breastfeeding": hence, the title of its manual. Many mothers have the idea that you should contact the League only if a problem arises. On the contrary, the League can be very valuable even to the successful nursing mother. La Leche League is represented by over a thousand groups located in many towns and cities throughout the United States and in other countries. The ideal time for a woman to complete the regular series of meetings given by the League is during pregnancy. The League's manual, *The Womanly Art of Breastfeeding*, is one book a nursing mother should have in her possession to read and reread when necessary.

NAPSAC International

This organization provides services in the area of pregnancy, childbirth and early infant care. Its book, *The Five Standards for Safe Childbearing*, is informative in the subjects of nutrition in pregnancy, natural childbirth, nursing your baby, and other topics important to expectant couples. The book is, in part, the edited transcripts of NAPSAC Conference presentations. Some readers may disagree with some of the speakers' content which is unrelated to the book's central theme — safe childbearing from conception through birth and breastfeeding. I mention this but still feel this book provides excellent, well documented and helpful information, much of which is not to be found in any other publication of which I am aware.

All of the above organizations publish informative newsletters. Contact the organizations for subscription rates; their addresses are in the front of this book. All three books, *The Womanly Art of Breastfeeding*, *The Five Standards for Safe Childbearing*, *The Art of Natural Family Planning*, and this book may be conveniently

100

purchased by mail through The Couple to Couple League. See mini-catalogue at the back of this book.

PERSONAL RECOMMENDATIONS

From my personal experience, I can offer several recommendations that may have wide applicability in helping mothers get off to a good start in breastfeeding after childbirth.

1. Read up on the subject. Reading helps you and your husband to become better informed. Your library may have some materials, but they may be far from equal in quality. Another problem with some childbirth books is that the authors may depart from their subject and suggest perverse sexual practices or they may refer to sources who dabble in witchcraft or the occult. Also, books change from one edition to another. Therefore I am not endorsing any particular book.

2. Express your feelings to the doctor and explain why you feel the way you do. Don't come armed with literature as if you expect a fight, but have your husband come with you for support.

Remember that you have the right to be selective in choosing your obstetrician, pediatrician, or family doctor. Exercise this right. Ask questions plainly. Having a list of important questions helps you to remember the things you wanted to ask. If a doctor has a set way of doing things, such as routine sonograms or routine fetal monitoring, don't be afraid to ask why. You have a right to refuse unnecessary treatment.

3. Be specific. Ask ahead of time whether you can have your baby with you after childbirth, whether you can have an unmedicated childbirth experience or at least a minimal amount of drugs if needed, whether you can totally nurse the baby for the first six months, and so forth.

4. You have a right to your own baby. He does not belong to the hospital.

5. You have a right to leave the hospital as soon as it is possible, consistent with the health of your baby and yourself.

6. You have a right to have the natural care that is best for you and your baby, and you can feel secure knowing that "science" is there for the unusual circumstance should you or the baby require special treatment.

7. Since "natural" in man does not mean the same as "automatic," you have a corresponding duty to prepare yourself ahead of time both intellectually and physically in order to fully assist the natural processes.

Don't expect a natural-type childbirth experience without childbirth preparation, and don't expect a successful nursing experience without learning something about breastfeeding. Make use of the services provided by childbirth education groups and by La Leche League and other nursing-mother groups.

8. Attend childbirth classes with each baby. The instructor we had when expecting our fourth child impressed me the most. She had several suggestions for specific situations and was not dogmatic and set into only one way of giving birth. Secondly, you still learn plus refresh your memory of what you once learned and may have forgotten. You also keep in touch with what's going on childbirth-wise if you are headed for a hospital birth.

9. You will also learn things from personal experience that you may not learn in the classroom. For example, I discovered labor ceases—for me—if I'm lying down. So I remain upright—sitting or standing—during most of labor; in this position progress is steady. I also found it comfortable to deliver upright as well and ended up in a squatting position with baby #4 and a kneeling position at the side of the bed with baby #5. My instructors did not tell me to do this. In fact, I had learned about delivering a baby in the lying down side position and thought I would try it, but lying down does not work for me. Under the circumstances you do what's "comfortable," and I was happy to have a doctor that encouraged this type of delivery.

10. Learn with your husband whenever possible. Share with him anything new that you've learned through contact with other nursing mothers or through reading. Go to the childbirth classes together.

11. You have a right to terminate your relationship with your doctor. If he won't go along with the best in maternal or pediatric care, don't feel you are obliged to stay with him; but find another one before you burn your bridges.

If you know that breastfeeding is best for your baby, if you know that a good start is important in the breastfeeding natural mothering relationship, if you know that obstetrical medication may have certain hazards for your baby and may impede early breastfeeding, then it seems to me that as an informed couple you would want to do everything reasonably possible to insure that the the childbirth experience will work to get the breastfeeding off to a good start and which will be the most healthy start for your baby.

To conclude, I would like to add that many of us who have breastfed owe a deep debt of gratitude to a particular doctor or nurse who gave us the proper support and advice with regard to childbirth and breastfeeding. It must also be realized that most hospitals and doctors practice as they do because that is what their patients want. Some mothers want to start their babies on solids right off the bat; some mothers want to be knocked out during the birth; some mothers tend to look to science to solve all their problems. There are doctors who would like to see a change, but they, too, are faced with the difficult job of reeducating their patients as to what is best for them. I know doctors who personally recommend breastfeeding or natural childbirth only to have many women turn up their noses. They just aren't interested.

Secondly, both the childbirth and the early breastfeeding experiences are interrelated and play an important part in the mother-baby ecology. If this ecology is greatly disturbed during childbirth and the immediate postpartum hours, then the breastfeeding and natural mothering relationship may be seriously hampered and even made almost impossible. I suggest that you read this chapter a second time and then take the necessary steps to make sure that your breastfeeding experience gets off to the best possible start.

References

1. The directory is available through NAPSAC, Box 646, Marble Hill, MO 63764.
2. Doris Haire, "The Cultural Warping of Childbirth," *ICEA News*, Spring 1972, p. 10.
3. "455,000 C-sections Called Unnecessary," *The Cincinnati Post*, November 2, 1987, p. 3A.
4. "Future babies," *U.S. News & World Report*, November 30, 1987, p. 72.
5. "Nature's Way May Be Better In Hard Births," *The Cincinnati Enquirer*, June 26, 1985, p. B-12.
6. Review of a ten minute film, "Birth in the Squatting Position," "Film Library," *Maternal Health News*, December 1988, p. 2.
7. Connie Livingston, "Okay, Honey, Push!" *Wet Set Gazette*, December 1988, p. 6.

10

The First Six Months

NATURE'S PRODUCT

Your milk is the best food you can give your baby. Breast milk has all the calories, proteins, vitamins, water, and other essential elements needed for your baby's growth—except Vitamin D which he makes from exposure to sunlight. Nature, which did a fantastic job of nurturing and developing new life within your body for nine months before birth, has likewise provided a complete nutritious food for your baby's growth after birth. Nature intends a continuity between the nourishment you gave your baby in your womb and the nourishment you can give your baby at your breasts. In fact, so great is this continuity that even if you should have a preterm baby, your milk is adjusted accordingly. "Several investigators have shown that the composition of preterm human milk may meet the nutritional needs of preterm infants better than term human milk."[1]

From the baby's point of view, unrestricted nursing from the very beginning may be quite important for his health. The secretion that comes from a mother's breast at birth, the colostrum, is different from and richer than the milk that will soon follow. This first milk is valuable to an infant's health, for cells present in colostrum ingest and destroy bacteria. The proportions of the constituents in human milk gradually change; the colostrum of the first day is not the same as the colostrum of the second, and no formula can duplicate these day by day and even hour by hour changes. When the transitional milk starts coming in, there are similar changes to meet the needs of the baby. Mother's milk is best for her baby right from the very beginning. Simple glucose or water is a poor substitute for the complex and rich initial diet the baby is entitled to receive from his mother's breast.

Breast milk contains an insufficient amount of Vitamin D, but apparently nature intended that both mother and baby obtain some Vitamin D out of doors, since our bodies synthesize this vitamin upon exposure to sunlight. Your doctor may or may not recommend vitamin drops for your breastfed baby. These drops will not influence the natural-spacing benefit derived from completely nursing your baby.

Breast milk contains a plentiful supply of Vitamin C when the mother's diet is adequate. This is evident when you observe any analytic breakdown of breast milk and its constituents. Therefore, juices that are often recommended in the baby's early months are unnecessary for the breastfed baby.

Some mothers are told to give their baby extra liquid or water during the hot summer months, but this is unnecessary. There is a sufficient amount of water in breast milk for the baby. If anyone needs the extra water, it would be the nursing mother herself. Therefore, for normal healthy infants, nature's complete food need not be supplemented with bottles containing juices, liquids, or plain water.

It should go without saying that a nursing mother should provide herself with good nutrition. The maternal diet is important in order for the baby to derive the greatest benefit from this ecological relationship. Therefore, during the months of pregnancy and during the months of breastfeeding a mother should take special care in selecting proper foods for herself and her family.

THE NEED FOR IRON

At birth the full-term baby has his own supply of iron which normally lasts until the time of weaning. This is especially true if the placenta has been allowed to detach naturally. If you plan to nurse your baby completely for six months or thereabouts, your doctor may want to check your baby's iron supply before he reaches six months of age. The testing is very simple and will cause little discomfort to your baby. A finger is pricked quickly to obtain a few drops of blood which is then measured. Many doctors today do not require any testing or iron supplementation if baby is healthy and solids are begun shortly after six months of age. The healthiness of this practice was demonstrated by a 1984 study in which the authors reported "that a great majority of exclusively breastfed infants are able to maintain their iron status at the same level as that of control infants receiving iron supplements;" and the authors noted they "could not demonstrate any anemia in infants after exclusive breastfeeding for 9 months." They concluded that their data "indicate that it is safe, in exclusively breastfed infants, to shift the starting age for iron supplementation to 6 months, or even older."[2]

SOLIDS—EARLY OR LATE?

The early introduction of solids is so common today that a mother who chooses to nurse her infant as the good Lord intended is rare indeed. Friends and relatives question her choice for fear her baby will become undernourished. For many, the saying "breastfed is best-fed," seems somehow unbelievable. They do not believe the baby will thrive unless there is something solid in its tummy.

Do babies thrive at the breast or not? Doctors are now questioning the practice of administering solids in the first four to six months. The Committee on Nutrition showed how the trend went from no solids during the first year of life before the 1920s and then switched gradually into a cultural practice of introducing solids during the first days of life. In their report in 1958, the committee (representing the American Academy of Pediatrics) stated that

. . .lacking is proof obtained from controlled observations that feeding of solid food at ages earlier than 4 to 6 months of life is nutritionally or psychologically beneficial or, on the other hand, is actually harmful. . .the feeding of solid foods nutritionally inferior to milk, at the expense of milk, could result in worsening the nutritional state of the infant rather than bettering it. . .No harmful results have been reported thus far, but potential danger exists that earlier supplementation of the milk diets of infants with solid food of inferior nutritional content may, because of satiety, result in a decreased intake of milk.[3]

What you will be seeing in the rest of this chapter is a series of reasons for delaying the introduction of solids for about six months. You will also see how the medical community, especially allergists and pediatricians, gradually came to this position—from the rather tentative 1958 statement above to a general acceptance thirty years later.

A 1974 report on infant nutrition in *The Lancet*, a highly regarded English medical journal, stressed 1) that breast milk up to the age of 4-6 months was preferable and 2) that early solids "are unnecessary and can be positively harmful." The report adds that

106

"the risks associated with bottle-feeding with cow's milk preparations—principally gastroenteritis and neonatal tetany—are particularly dangerous in the first weeks of life, and breastfeeding for even 2 weeks can be advantageous."[4]

Another factor that contributes to the early solids rush is our excessive concern for the baby's weight. More weight seems to be equated with better health. But is a fat baby necessarily a healthy baby? Back in 1958 Dr. Gilbert Forbes questioned the early introduction of solids for which there is no proven need.[5] In a popular women's magazine, Stanley Englebardt demonstrated through research and various medical opinions that overweight in an infant can lead to obesity in later life. Early overfeeding means the formation of more fat cells, cells a person keeps throughout his entire lifetime. Because of these additional fat cells, a fat baby will have greater difficulty staying slim in later years. He quoted several doctors who agreed that prevention of obesity begins in infancy, a time when eating habits are formed. One of the doctors he quoted, Dr. Virginia Vivian, a nutritionist from Ohio State University, stated that the first six months may be the most crucial in determining the number of fat cells.[6]

Totally breastfed babies can appear obese as babies. However, a physician friend of ours who has seen many obese babies—breastfed and bottle-fed—says that there is a difference when they become toddlers and begin walking and running. He claims the bottle-fed youngster tends to retain his heaviness while the breastfed youngster slims down in appearance.

The early feeding of solids does not appear to have any rational basis, except that parents hope solids will help their babies go longer between feedings and help them sleep through the night. Other reasons given for the early introduction of solids or supplementation are 1) the advertisements in lay and professional magazines, 2) the insistence of mothers or of doctors, and 3) the easy availability of baby cereals, pureed foods, and formulas.

OTHER REASONS FOR WAITING

There is no question that many more American women are nursing their newborns in the late eighties than in the sixties. Much of this undoubtedly mirrors the increased health concerns of Western culture in general during the same years. However, some mothers may be unaware of all the specific advantages of breastfeeding. What follows will offer you encouragement and conviction in your desire to nurse your baby.

1. **Babies do gain well on breast milk alone.** Mothers often doubt this fact until they see it for themselves. One mother wrote, "I laugh now when I think of how I asked John if your babies were healthy and if they gained weight just nursing." Some mothers become concerned because their baby did not gain much by the first monthly visit, but even these mothers become confident as they observe with pride their growing breastfed baby.

A 1964 study on weight gain was carefully conducted by several doctors and involved some 599 babies who were under observation for one year. A select group of 89 babies were completely nursed for six months (no vitamins and no solids were administered). Breast milk was their only intake. No signs of rickets or anemia were observed in this group of babies, even though no other source of Vitamin D or iron was administered in the first six months of life and these babies were outside only during the warmer months of the year. The doctors found that this group of babies grew at the same rate as the other two groups of babies under observation: 1) infants who were completely nursed for six months and received vitamin supplements and 2) infants who were bottle-fed and received vitamin supplements.[7]

2. **Breastfed babies are healthier.** Dr. Robbins Kimball has observed that during the first ten years of life the breastfed youngster is healthier and is more resistant to infections than a bottle-fed child. The bottle-fed child has "4 times the respiratory infections, 20 times the diarrhea, 22 times the miscellaneous infections, 8 times the eczema, 21 times the asthma, 27 times the hayfever," and he also had eleven times more tonsilectomies and four times more ear infections. In his study he also found the bottle-fed child had "11 times the hospital admissions and 8 times the house calls."[8]

Dr. Richard Applebaum in his book, *Abreast of the Times*, stresses the health benefits from colostrum by stating that this first milk 1) contains "natural antibodies against measles, polio, mumps and a host of other diseases;" 2) acts on a bacteria *(E. coli)* that "is notorious for causing infant diarrhea the first month of life" and may cause infantile meningitis; and 3) offers the baby "protection against respiratory infections, such as flu and pneumonia." During one cold winter he observed that of the babies who were brought into his office for colds, coughs, and high fevers, none were breastfed.[9]

While we lived in California our pediatrician was also impressed with the health of the breastfed babies in his practice. This impression left him with the desire to learn more about breastfeeding as he admitted having learned very little about it in medical school. He observed in his own work that the overall health of the breastfed baby was superior to the overall health of the bottle-fed baby.

Jelliffe and Jelliffe conclude that "cow's milk preparations have no scientific advantage or superiority over human milk." The only advantage of a cow's milk preparation, as they see it, is its usefulness for the working mother. Indeed, in some areas of the world, breast milk is a nutritional necessity for maintaining a healthy infant. From the research they conclude:

In less technically developed areas of the world, including underprivileged groups in industrialized countries, the antidiarrheal and nutrition importance of breastfeeding is increasingly obvious as the sole food for 4 to 6 months and as a small, but significant, protein supplement thereafter during the first two or more years of life. Ironically, at the same time, the disastrous trend to unaffordable artificial feeding continues in peri-urban areas, with increasing prevalence of marasmus and diarrhea in early infancy, a period of high vulnerability for immediate ill effects and long-term damage.[10]

At the Ninth International Congress of Nutrition, the consensus among the doctors was that breast milk alone should be offered during the baby's first three to four months and that "supplements, solids, or other milk should not be fed until the first three or four months under any circumstances except emergencies." The doctors said that breast milk protects a child from obesity, diarrhea, staph, and other infections. Regarding obesity: "The bottle-fed baby is highly susceptible to multi-cell obesity, a condition in which cells develop which retain fat even in the face of rigorous weight control efforts. Early feeding of solid foods compounds this problem, in the opinion of Dr. D. B. Jelliffe, professor of pediatrics and public health at the University of California at Los Angeles."[11]

Companies which manufacture baby foods have been severely criticized for adding unnecessary items to the jar's contents that may be harmful to the infant's health—namely, too much sugar, salt, and starch. Of course, a mother who follows the natural inclinations of her child would not be bothered with buying special baby foods. Breast milk suffices until the baby begins to help himself from the table.

Many of us have been acquainted with babies who require special formulas which can be quite costly. This expense, of course, could have been avoided if the mother had been breastfeeding in the first place. There are also a few babies who would have died if breast milk had not been available to them. I would like to quote from two letters I received while in the process of writing this book.

Our league here has just had a rewarding experience in providing breast-milk for a very premature baby who could not tolerate formula and [his condition] was becoming very critical. The pediatrician called La Leche League as a last resort as the mother was not nursing. After being given breastmilk, the baby improved immediately and surpassed his birthweight of slightly over two pounds.

Right now we are supplying a baby with breast milk. He was three and a half months old and barely living at eight pounds in the University Hospital at Saskatoon when I was asked if we could provide breast milk for him. Now (a month later) he is a healthy eleven pounds fourteen ounces and growing at an unbelievable rate. The mother is trying to relactate but is having quite a bit of difficulty. . .There is no doubt that this baby would have died had he not gotten breast milk.

3. **Breastfed babies develop fewer allergies.** Dr. Frank Richardson, author of *The Nursing Mother*, noted that

delaying the addition of solid or semisolid foods until the baby is five or six months old does no harm; and giving them earlier probably serves no specially valuable purpose. . .Furthermore, the allergists are almost unanimous in asserting that the earlier solid foods are introduced, the more likely a child is to become sensitized to them.[12]

Doctors Jerome Glaser and Eric M. Dreyfuss note that "Breast-feeding is the most important single measure in the prophylaxis [prevention] of allergic disease."[13] And Dr. Paul Gyorgy, a pediatrician who received the American Pediatric Society's annual Howland Award in 1968 for distinguished achievement, discouraged the early introduction of solids or supplements because these foods are the leading allergens among infants.[14]

In a review article about allergy to cow's milk, Doctors N. W. Wilson and R. N. Hamburger noted that between 2 percent and 3 percent of the general population of infants are allergic to cow's milk but that such allergy may reach the 30 percent level among children who inherit allergic tendencies from their parents. The treatment is common sense: "Avoidance [of cow's milk] is the mainstay of treatment and breastfeeding is the optimal choice," and that means "exclusive breastfeeding for about 6 months combined with delayed introduction to solid foods for at least 6 months."[15] This is especially necessary for those with inherited allergic tendencies but makes good sense for all.

Breastfed babies also have less diaper rash. Mothers who have bottle-fed previous babies and then switched to breastfeeding for a later baby have found that the breastfed baby requires less care. These mothers have found that they can use plastic pants, change cloth diapers at longer intervals, and only occasionally dip into the Vaseline jar. By comparison, with previous babies they went through jar after jar of Vaseline and had to change diapers more frequently.

4. **Breastfeeding saves kitchen time.** Time that isn't spent in the kitchen preparing bottles, nipples, and formula or spent in cleaning up afterwards is time better spent with baby. Breastfeeding means food for the baby that takes no time to prepare and only a little time to serve. It's even quicker than an "instant breakfast," but who's in a rush anyway? The food is ready any time or anywhere for the asking and is always at the right temperature. There is no need to warm it up or cool it down. Instead of work, it means "little breaks" during the day to sit down (or lie down) and enjoy the children God gave you.

Breastfeeding generally means fewer visits to the doctor or hospital. It means less work for a sick mother who can care for her baby in bed. It may mean less work for the physically handicapped mother who would also enjoy this intimate contact with her baby. It means one hand free to hug a child, answer the phone, or eat a meal.

Breastfeeding means carefree traveling with no special baby stops, whether it's a day outing for the family, a week's vacation or a trip to Europe. For campers, it's the best way to travel with a baby.

5. **Breastfeeding saves money.** Money not spent on bottles, nipples, brushes, sterilizer, formula, juice, foods, food and bottle warmers, and the gas or electricity required in the preparation is money saved. In the years to come it usually means less money spent on doctors' fees, hospital expenses, and probably fewer drugs and fewer dental bills. Breastfeeding costs nothing except tender loving care.

Nursing mothers have figured out that when a mother nurses her baby completely for the entire first six months, the savings easily add up to enough to buy a basic king-size or queen-size bed—which I suggest that you do. It makes sleeping with your baby much easier.

6. **Nature has a diet plan for your baby.** The presence of a strong sucking reflex and the absence of teeth are physical signs indicating that nature intended babies to have milk in the first months of life. Later, some physical changes occur. The teeth begin to come in at a very slow pace, and the swallowing reflex has developed. Baby has already started manipulating anything he

can grasp toward his mouth. All of these changes suggest that baby will soon be ready to take food off the table. The Committee on Nutrition has said that the

rooting and sucking reflex exhibited in the newborn, and persisting for many months, would indicate that this is the normal method by which the infant obtains food. . .Salivary secretion, as manifested by drooling, usually does not make its appearance until the third or fourth month. Teeth appear around 6 months of age and chewing motions are a later accomplishment. All of these are indicative of nature's plan for a liquid diet for the first few months of life.[16]

The general reaction of babies to early solids was studied by Virginia Beal of the Child Research Council. "The most common picture is one of eagerness for the bottle but resistance to feeding of other foods, with crying or fussing or spitting out, until a time, usually between 4 or 6 months of age, when the child begins to accept willingly the solid foods."[17]

Even when babies are good eaters at one or two months of age, mothers still say that it's a lot of unnecessary bother. And besides, it usually means giving him less and less of the best food which you alone can offer him.

7. **Baby and mother thrive on each other.** The emotional benefits of breastfeeding are valued as highly as the physical benefits by many doctors and experts today. More and more emphasis is being placed on the importance of skin-to-skin contact between parent and child—whether it be in the act of nursing a baby, rubbing a child's back, or rocking a child to sleep. Physical contact generates warm feelings of being loved and appreciated. Breastfeeding guarantees the child frequent contact with his mother. Dr. Grantly Dick-Read has written:

What are three things these children require and thrive on? 1) They are born to seek food at once from the mother's breast. . .2) They desire warmth from the mother's body. And then, perhaps what is more important, 3) they need security in their mother's presence. These three factors are the only provision that nature demands all children should have for their first weeks of neonatal life. Breastfeeding satisfies all three.[18]

The emotional benefits flowing from the breastfeeding act are just as important to the mother. Breastfeeding is a very satisfying and enjoyable experience for the nursing mother. It grows on her, and she seems to enjoy it more as the baby grows older and as she has other babies. This is probably the main reason why many mothers are so enthusiastic about nursing. Breastfeeding, I am

112

convinced, helps the mother to thrive as a mother. And we have already seen how breastfeeding helps the baby to thrive.

It seems fitting to close this chapter with another quotation from Doctors Glaser and Dreyfuss:

The superiority of breast milk as compared with cow's milk has never been questioned. It is too often forgotten that breast milk is the only natural food for the human infant, at least during the first few months of life.[19]

References

1. Edward A. Liechty, "Nutrition in the Premature Infant," *Practice of Pediatrics*, V.C. Kelley, ed. (Philadelphia: Harper and Row, 1987), Vol.6, Chapter 18, p. 14.
2. Martti A. Siimes et al, "Exclusive breastfeeding for nine months: risk of iron deficiency," *Journal of Pediatrics* 104:2(1984)199.
3. Committee on Nutrition, "On the Feeding of Solid Foods to Infants," *Pediatrics* 21:4(April 1958)685-692.
4. "Breastfeeding Is Best," *The Lancet* 2(October 26, 1974)1029.
5. Gilbert Forbes, "Do We Need a New Perspective in Infant Nutrition?" *Journal of Pediatrics* 52(1958)496.
6. Stanley Englebardt, "Are You Overfeeding Your Child?" *Woman's Day*, July 1971, p. 12.
7. R.L. Jackson et al., "Growth of 'Well-born' American Infants Fed Human and Cow's Milk," *Pediatrics* 33(1964)642.
8. Robbins E. Kimball, "How I Get Mothers to Breastfeed," *Physician's Management*, June 1968.
9. Richard Applebaum, *Abreast of the Times* (Privately published, 1969) p. 11.
10. D.B. Jelliffe and E.F.P. Jelliffe, "The Uniqueness of Human Milk," *The American Journal of Clinical Nutrition*, 24(August 1971)1019.
11. "Cow's Milk—Not As Good For Baby As Mother's Own," *The Cincinnati Enquirer*, September 9, 1972, p. 12.
12. Frank Richardson, *The Nursing Mother*, (Englewood Cliffs: Prentice-Hall, 1953) p. 141.
13. Jerome Glaser and Eric M. Dreyfuss, "Prenatal and Postnatal Prophylaxis of Allergic Disease," *Practice of Pediatrics,* V.C. Kelley, ed., (Philadelphia: Harper and Row, 1982) Vol.2, Chapter 89, p. 7.
14. Paul Gyorgy, "Trends and Advances in Infant Nutrition," *The West Virginia Medical Journal* 53:4(April 1957)131-138.
15. Nevin W. Wilson and Robert N. Hamburger, "Allergy to cow's milk in the first year of life and its prevention," *Annals of Allergy* 61:5(November 1988)323-327.
16. Committee on Nutrition, *op. cit.*, p. 690.
17. Virginia Beal, "On the Acceptance of Solid Foods, and Other Food Patterns, of Infants and Children," *Pediatrics* 20(1957)448.
18. Grantly Dick-Read, *Childbirth Without Fear,* 4th Edition (New York: Harper & Row, 1972) p. 92.
19. Glaser and Dreyfuss, *loc. cit.*

11

Nursing the Older Child

NATURE'S NORM

Experience has shown that the mother who follows this book's pattern of natural mothering will usually be nursing well beyond her baby's first birthday. In our first survey of breastfeeding and amenorrhea, the group that followed this pattern averaged 14.6 months of amenorrhea with continued nursing and averaged almost 23.0 months of breastfeeding. Over 40 percent nursed beyond the child's second birthday, and a few went close to and even beyond the third birthday. Thus it is evident that some normal American women are experiencing the same kind of extended natural mothering pattern that is common in cultures that are very much in touch with nature. In this chapter we will use the term "older child" to refer to the baby who has passed his first birthday, and we'll be looking at some reasons for nursing the older child, some cultural attitudes, and some ways for the long-term nursing mother to find support when some of the other gals tell her she's a nut.

In our culture it is expected that a baby will be weaned from the breast at least by ten months of age or by the time he begins to walk. The nine- or ten-month period following childbirth is a common time for nursing mothers to wean. In our first survey, out of the entire group, 25.0 percent weaned between nine and twelve months (the most common time in our survey), and 20.6 percent weaned between thirteen and sixteen months (the next most common time). This, keep in mind, was from a group of women interested enough in breastfeeding to have read the first, privately published edition of this book.

It must be remembered that people are not used to hearing of women who nurse longer than a year, and that secondly, most people have a very limited view of breastfeeding. There are those who look at breastfeeding only in terms of nutrition or those who see it only as a means of birth control. If you look at breastfeeding primarily or even exclusively as a way of satisfying baby's hunger pains, then you can readily see why a baby could be weaned by ten months. With the introduction of solids and early use of the cup, breastfeeding is no longer necessary except for medical reasons (e.g., allergies). And, for those who look upon breastfeeding primarily as a means of avoiding a pregnancy, once menstruation resumes there is no reason to continue the nursing relationship. Moreover, even some of those who are most adamant about breastfeeding in the early months for the full range of nutritional and emotional reasons are either shocked or surprised to learn that a mother is nursing an older child. On the other hand, if breastfeeding involves a whole method of child care and if the breast is looked upon as a wonderful mothering tool, then there is no need to have a cut-off date. A mother may as well take advantage of this easy form of mothering while she can. Two or three years of nursing may sound like a long time, but in terms of the child's lifetime it is brief.

Unfortunately, some people will find cruel explanations for prolonged nursing. They may say that the mother is smothering the child or that she is nursing for sexual kicks. Some will infer that she is using the baby as a birth-control device. They will worry that the mother is being neglectful or that the baby will be psychologically damaged. Will the baby boy grow up to be effeminate or will the child have homosexual tendencies? Is the baby addicted to the breast? The above fears are unfounded. In fact, the widely publicized apparent increase in homosexuality occurs in an age of bottle-feeding and early weaning practices. Certainly, prolonged breastfeeding is not accountable in our society for this incidence. In the light of the severely critical comments that are sometimes made, it is helpful to have the support of others when you are nursing the child according to his own timetable for nursing.

NURSING NEEDS OF THE OLDER CHILD

Maria Montessori supports nature's guidelines for mothering. Her views about early infant care are well expressed in *The Absorbent Mind*. She advises parents to respect the child's natural development. "Localized states of maturity must first be established, and the effort to force the child's natural development can only do harm. It is nature that directs. Everything depends on her and must obey her command."[1]

Once a mother has decided to go along with her baby and let him wean himself at his own pace, she may have some second thoughts. Perhaps she thought this meant a couple of extra months—and now he's almost two. Could he possibly still have a need for breastfeeding? Interestingly enough, we see nothing strange in a two-year-old using a bottle or a pacifier. However, because the long-term nursing mother is an exception in our culture, the doubts persist. She can take comfort in these passages from Eda LeShan's *How Do Your Children Grow?*

We also have to understand, and this holds true all through parenthood, that when a need is met, it goes away. Children of any age do not continue to behave in certain ways unless there is a need. When they are finished with it, they will give it up. Sometimes it may go on longer than we expect, and a parent will worry because a sixteen-month-old is still nursing. This is a very natural tendency. We think the things that are happening will go on forever. The truth is that they will go on only as they are needed.[2]

However, we worry far too much about the need lasting too long. That is less likely to do any damage than the opposite, cutting it off too quickly. The one thing that upsets parents and children more than anything else is the unfinished business of any one phase of life. If a child needs to go through some kind of an emotional experience, and he doesn't go through it at the time that is most appropriate, it is never finished, according to LeShan.[3]

Prolonged breastfeeding may also prove helpful in emergency situations or during an illness. Temporary emergency situations, such as car trouble or bad weather conditions, may cause a period of isolation during which nursing would be advantageous. Prolonged breastfeeding may influence your baby's health even after his first birthday. The older baby who loses his appetite during an illness will at least receive good nourishment from the breast at a time when he might not take any other foods. Here is a story of one mother who was grateful that she had continued to nurse her child:

When our second son was being seen by his pediatrician for his first yearly checkup, the doctor questioned me about his still being nursed. "Aren't you ever going to wean him? You know, he's not needing this physically for nutrition anymore." I answered, "Great! I'll go home with a pacified doctor and a very frustrated baby." We both laughed and I assured the doctor that he would wean—but at **his** own rate.

Two months later the baby became ill with an intestinal virus. His fever was 105 and we rushed him to the hospital. For two days and nights he was kept on clear liquids and nursing. Even with this, the diarrhea was so severe that the doctor ordered IV's to prevent further dehydration. This lasted forty-eight hours. During this period I couldn't even nurse him. Actually, he was so sick that he slept most of the time—so I was the one who suffered with full breasts.

Hand expressing and pumping with the breast pump somehow just didn't seem to empty my breasts as completely as a baby nursing does. I'm certain that a good deal of it was psychological for me, too. By the end of the second day the doctor asked me, "Do you think he still remembers how to nurse after this long? If he does and **since** it's breast milk—I'll let him have the milk. I know he'll regain his strength faster. Also it won't upset his intestines like 'foreign' milk would." Still remember how? You don't practice something several times a day for fourteen months and then forget in two days! I only wish I had words to describe how eagerly he settled against me—knowing **exactly** where he was going. Joy and relief flooded us both!

Later during a visit to the doctor's office, the pediatrician gave me one of the nicest compliments I ever had with a nursing experience: "You've shown me how important it is to follow a baby-led weaning pattern, and never will I pressure a mother about weaning again."

The most common reason given for prolonged breastfeeding is the special relationship that a mother has with her child. This closeness is strengthened over a period of two or three years through the nursing relationship, and it cannot easily be lost once the breastfeeding comes to an end. The bond is still there, and a mother can maintain it through other avenues of affection and communication, physical or verbal. One wonders whether the "generation gap" begins at such an early time. Would more parents be in tune with their children if they had breastfed for a considerable length of time? Would children be more sensitive to their parents' feelings if they had experienced this long-term relationship with the one parent in early childhood?

Certainly there are other factors that can influence our relationships with our children, but today we parents need all the help we can get to do a better job of raising our children. We also need easier methods, and breastfeeding at least makes the job easier during those early years. Whether it helps in later years is speculative. Other parents have told us there is a bond and closeness with their breastfed child that they didn't achieve when they bottle-fed. This closeness has also matured them and given them a deeper appreciation of the needs of their older children and even of other children in the immediate neighborhood.

The warm relationship that develops during the first years as

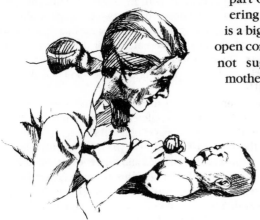

part of the natural mothering program certainly is a big help in developing open communications. I am not suggesting that the mother who lets her children breastfeed into the second, third, or fourth year will have no communication problems with them in the teen years. What I am suggesting, however, is that the close relationship and the habit of being open to the young child's needs provide an excellent start. The parents who maintain this habit of openness to the child's needs should have less difficulty during those adolescent years. One mother wrote:

My second oldest child was fifteen yesterday. As I look back as I have done repeatedly in the last ten years since my joy of discovering breastfeeding, I'm still regretful about those years of bottle-feeding with my first three children. It is said that you don't cry over spilled milk, but I do, and I think that is my underlying motivation in trying to help other mothers and families.

We have all heard various psychologists say something to the effect that a child's character or the way he will respond to different situations is pretty much set by the time he enters kindergarten. If during a good half of those years he found security and warmth at his mother's breast, as he needed it and not as someone else dictated, then this would seem to be a good foundation of trust for the later years.

However, keep this in mind: breastfed Cain slew breastfed Abel. In other words, a long and strong breastfeeding relationship is no guarantee that problems will not develop later. However, the relationship developed then and continued through full-time mothering may reduce the extent of later problems.

Regardless of what the future holds, the fact still remains that as parents of young children we are called to respond to their needs with ourselves and not just with things that money can buy. Doing our best for the child, giving him the best of everything doesn't mean only clothes, schools, toys, transportation, vacations, lessons, tutors, baby-sitters, and money. As Dr. James L. Hymes, Jr., tells us in *The Child Under Six*, "One way or another adults must help themselves to realize what is our adult job—to give to children. Not things, but ourselves. We give our time, our love, our care. Babies cannot do for themselves. We have to be on hand, gladly, to meet their needs."[4]

There is no doubt that while natural mothering at times is more convenient than using artifacts, it also takes time. Best of all, it always gives individual attention, which may be looked upon as a wise investment in the child's future. Margaret Mead, in an excellent article, "Working Mothers and Their Children," expressed concern over the type of care the young child receives in day care centers: "Only individual attention can turn a child into a full human being, capable of growth." She criticized a frequent change in the mother-figure and noted that a small child "needs someone who is intensely interested in him or her, who will spend endless hours responding and initiating, repeating sounds, noting nuances of expression, reinforcing new skills, bolstering self-confidence and a sense of self." A child who receives such continuity, she claims, "can survive a great many changes of place and person later." Persons who have not had such care "have less capacity to trust the world, to leave home happily, and to form wider and more intense relationships with other people later."[5] Considering the many changes of place and persons that some children experience in our mobile society, the individual time and attention spent in natural mothering is a sound investment.

I think there are other benefits of prolonged nursing that lets the child wean at his own pace. Natural breastfeeding helps the parent to accept the child for what he is. Instead of imposing outside norms, natural mothering looks to the inner growth pattern of the child. The child's growth in all its phases is specially guarded and respected. These phases of growth are not forced to end too early, nor are they forced to remain when the need is no longer present. This acceptance and love for the child as he is may help the parents to accept him at his own level of interests and development in later years.

Another tremendous benefit from prolonged breastfeeding is the stimulation that the child receives when his mother takes him with her. He is exposed to a wide variety of social circumstances and, in addition, he has the security of his parents or his mother wherever he goes. This stimulation is probably far greater than that which he would receive by remaining at home with sitters.

By no means least among the benefits of prolonged nursing is the continuation of family-centeredness. In the family where ecological breastfeeding is used in the first year, the baby is always a part of the family: the parents don't take off and leave him. Likewise when the mother continues to let her baby nurse beyond the first year, she will not be leaving him for extended periods of time. Instead, she will want to be near him, and she and her husband will plan recreational activities that are family oriented. The child who grows up in such a family today is lucky indeed. Family life in America is such that professionals are becoming concerned; it is too common for parents to look upon children as a burden or as second-class citizens within the family; the parents are constantly striving to get away from their children. The extended nursing of natural mothering is a tendency in the other direction.

SOME CHARACTERISTICS OF THE OLDER NURSING CHILD

What can you expect from the older nursing child? First, you will find that your child will ask for the breast at any time or place. In fact, he may ask for it at a time when you do not want him to ask, when you are around strangers or new relatives and friends. This presents a new environment to the child, and, in looking for security from his mother, he often seeks it at the breast.

You can avoid some embarrassment for yourself by having the child call the breast "ma-ma" or "mum-mum" or any word other than that which resembles a word like "nursie." You may also not call it anything: your child will simply inform you of his intentions by pulling or tugging at your top. If other persons are around, they will probably not pick up the clue. You can leave temporarily to nurse or explain the situation to the company or hostess. If you are away from home, the hostess can lead you into a more secluded area, such as her bedroom or den.

Of course, under some circumstances you could nurse on the spot without offending people or feeling funny, but such situations are rare today. You will also find that it is harder to nurse modestly with a bigger baby. He is too big for blankets; thus, the blanket can't be used as a shield. There is also a good chance he will dislike clothing too close to his face. He may pull at your bra or clothing in a playful manner, so that attention is actually drawn toward the nursing area. An older child may touch or lay his hand on the other breast while nursing, and this may offend people. Considering the situation, it is usually best to nurse only among those who understand and appreciate this type of mothering.

You will note other changes as you nurse the older child. He is talkative, playful, and affectionate. His responses are greatly varied. At times he will even tell you where to nurse him! There is also more give and take. He can appreciate the fact that you are busy, and he can wait a few minutes for a nursing. He can also learn to wait that one hour during church service, especially as he gets older.

You can also expect nursing sprees. Some days you will wonder why your child wants to nurse every hour for a few minutes or why the child wants to nurse almost continuously during the night. We noticed, for example, that after we moved to another state our three-year-old nursed almost constantly during the night for several weeks. Sometimes it can be explained and other times it can't be explained, but trust that this will pass in due time and the child will reduce the frequency.

As your child reaches the age of two or three years, you will find that he will not want to nurse in front of others who are strange to him. He will prefer to nurse only in front of family members. He may not want his parents or brothers and sisters to discuss his nursing with others in his presence or to tattle to his friends. His wishes should be respected within the family.

You may also find that your child is still nursing frequently in spite of being older. In writing and talking with other mothers, I find that it is common for older children reaching their second or even third birthday to be nursing quite frequently still. Some people feel that if a child has other brothers or sisters to keep him busy, or if a mother keeps her child interested in other activities, the child will lose interest in the breast. I find little support for this view. In the busiest of households and with mothers who stimulate their youngsters toward various activities, the child will still take the time to nurse in the midst of it all.

Night feedings can be expected while your older child is still nursing. In our study of mothers who nursed in a manner similar to the natural mothering program, most mothers nursed for as many months as they gave night feedings. They averaged almost twenty- four months of night feedings: the real average would be an even longer time, since a little over 50 percent were still giving night feedings at the time of the survey. Usually the last feedings to be dropped are those related to sleep. Therefore, toward the end of his nursing career the child will be nursing before naptime or before bedtime in the evening. If this situation does happen, then no one except your husband will know that your child is still nursing—unless you tell them. His last feeding may occur in the middle of the night.

An older nursing baby can begin to take brief separations from mom, such as an hour or two at the most, especially if he is having a good time at home or if he has a person caring for him that he likes. These brief separations can begin somewhere after the child's first birthday, but the time varies when a child accepts these separations of an hour or two willingly.

Daytime or early evening separations are easier for the child to accept. Upon your return you may find the babysitter or your husband telling you that your child was just beginning to miss you and was asking about you. Our last two children experienced their first separation at 15 and 18 months respectively. The occasion was their parents' decision to have dinner out alone. The fifteen-month-old started missing me before I returned; the eighteen-month-old hardly knew I had left. When I left the latter child the first time for a full day when he was five, he weathered the day with no upset. However, for the next few days, he would scarcely let me out of his sight.

I don't want mothers to set any goals by my babies, nor do I want to have mothers feel guilty for leaving their children at home. I mention this only because I've been told of mothers who so misinterpreted what I've written elsewhere that they felt guilty because of leaving a two-year-old home for a short time. You and your child can communicate and work these things out together. If you try a brief separation sometime and it doesn't work out, then wait a while before you try another. Once separations do begin, they should be infrequent at first with a lot of consideration given to the child.

Nighttime separations can be much harder for a child under two years of age. A child who has been nursed as described in this book may at 18 months choose to stay home with dad while mother runs to the store during the daytime. But this same child may have a strong need to be near mother at night. We accepted this fact, mainly from past experiences, and took our younger children with us everywhere in the evenings (be it social, for meetings, or for classes which we taught) for their first two years of life. When they turned two, after a few explanations and discussions, each child would decide he or she was big enough to stay home for the two or three hours we would be gone. Even then, we would occasionally come home to a child staring out the window waiting for our return.

Nighttime separations are easier to handle when the older children are understanding of the situation and are therefore very helpful or the babysitter is compassionate and is willing to hold the child a lot, read to him, etc. If one nighttime separation is hard on your child, then bring him with you the next time. Most two-year-olds soon learn how boring adult company and meetings are and decide to stay home at nights on their own.

Sometimes bringing a baby sitter along with you and your child or children is a good alternative to separation. For example, when our children were two, four and six years old, we played tennis at a park where the playground area was across a busy street opposite the courts. So we hired an older girl in the neighborhood to come and watch the children at the park. This way we all had a good time.

We found a similar solution while teaching natural family planning classes. Our fourth child was content to remain near me during our two hour classes, but our fifth child was very active and into everything. So, his sisters took turns coming to class to baby-sit him while we taught. His sisters knew he needed to be near me and so this arrangement worked well for us.

Overnight and weekend separations can be hard on young children. In a question-and-answer session following a talk in Cincinnati, Dr. Marshall Klaus, co-author of *Maternal-Infant Bonding*, was asked at what age would it be all right for the parents to leave their child for an overnight or weekend trip. He answered he would advise parents to wait until the child was at least four or five years old and then the parents should call their child the night or each night of their absence. This call would be reassuring to the child that mom and dad are doing fine.

Many separation decisions will be based on the communication you have with your child, the feelings you both have about separation, and who will be taking care of your child or children. It's one thing if its grandparents or other relatives with whom your children have a close rapport. It's something else to hire a live-in baby-sitter. And at the bottom of the pit, in the opinion of my husband who experienced it at about age six or seven, is placing your children in a boarding "academy" if such things still exist.

In summary, there seem to be four factors related to non-traumatic separations—age of the child, length of separation, frequency of separation, and your temporary mother-substitute. Wait till your child is ready. Then by making your initial separations short, you build up trust; just about the time he starts to miss you, you're home. Make your separations infrequent; children generally do not like their parents—especially both parents—out of the home several nights a week. And have as much consistency as you can in hiring a baby-sitter if one is needed.

FINAL WEANING

In natural mothering the time of final weaning is unpredictable because it is at the child's own pace. Sometimes a mother expects to nurse a baby for about two years only to be surprised to find that her child weans much earlier. Such a mother must realize that mothering isn't limited to the breast but that there are other ways to meet his needs. She can still provide body contact and lots of love and do many things with him. She can be assured that she satisfied his needs at the breast. On the other hand, there are other children who will be on only a few nursings a day for a long period of time before they gradually lose interest. A few mothers may feel guilty that their child doesn't nurse as frequently as Mrs. Jones's baby, and they'll be disappointed when their baby refuses the breast. I think the main point to remember is to enjoy your baby and **his** schedule. Contented mothering is the goal, not competitive mothering.

THE EXAMPLE OF OTHERS

Despite the many benefits that mothers have found to be associated with the extended nursing of natural mothering, it is still a difficult thing to consider in our culture. Most people will not appreciate long-term nursing unless they have done it, have known a close friend or relative who has done it, or have found themselves in the situation where it was evident that their baby still desired to be at the breast. The desire to nurse an older baby often comes by way of example. A mother can be encouraged to continue nursing her child if she knows of another mother who is nursing an older baby. Other mothers have wanted to nurse longer but quit because they knew of no one else who was doing it.

Your own feelings about nursing the older child will change as your nursing experience develops or matures with age. Reasons for prolonged lactation will probably play a small part in this change of attitudes. What will change your feelings on the subject at the time will be that one-year-old or two-year-old in your arms who still needs you. The pressures from society to wean may encourage you to stall a feeding only to find tears rolling down your child's cheeks—and you lovingly take him to breast. Secondly, the relationship is too enjoyable for its ending to be hastened, so you will find yourself learning to appreciate a new dimension in it.

How can you handle the reaction of others with respect to long-range nursing? First of all, you can appreciate why others feel the way they do about prolonged nursing when you try to picture somebody else's two- or three-year-old still nursing. I have nursed an older child—my own—yet it's always a surprise to hear that another older child that I know is still nursing. Having been there, I can appreciate that type of long-term nursing, but not many parents in our culture have had this experience, even though their numbers are gradually increasing. What makes the difference in one's feeling with regard to the older age is the fact that this is your child. There is a special relationship that you would want to have only with your child.

You should also realize that the relative infrequency of long-term nursing is in itself a cause of unfavorable reactions. Some people are unfavorably impressed by almost anything out of the ordinary, and a great number of otherwise well-educated people are simply amazed to learn that a mother can still be producing milk two and three years after childbirth.

Because your audience will most likely think you're crazy, there's no reason in the world why you have to volunteer information. Don't tell them that you are still nursing if you don't have to. If a situation develops where you find you have to tell, my husband and I have found that the best policy in handling other persons' questions is usually to be honest and "sure-headed." You will discover that there is very little static or none at all when you convey the attitude that you are confident in what you are doing and that you feel that this is the way it should be done. If you don't like to give personal reasons, you can always refer to women in other parts of the world and to those American women who nursed for several years before the "bottle" generations. Other mothers have found it extremely helpful to throw the attention to another nursing mother by saying, "I have a friend who is nursing a child who is even older than ours." If you do know of someone who is nursing a child older than yours, you will find that this offers you a great deal of support. The best support a nursing mother can have, however, is her husband. If her husband is 100 percent behind her, then an unkind remark will not hurt nearly as badly. It is wonderful to have a husband step in and handle the discussion, especially when the reactions are quite strong.

In the last analysis, if you are engaged in prolonged nursing because your child still wants to nurse and not out of some personal whim "to show the world" or to compete with somebody else, if you recognize that this is common in many cultures of the world, and if your husband supports you, then you have nothing to fear. On the other hand, you should not look down on the mother who is engaged in the child care typical of American culture. Ignorance is usually the greatest barrier to freedom. A person can't choose something before she knows about it, and most American women have never been exposed to the ideas we call natural mothering.

Today we hear much talk about changing life styles, some of which concerns a return to nature. This doesn't mean that we have to move out of the city or that everybody has to have an organic garden. Nature isn't to be found just in the fields and the forest or among the animals. Though our nature is incomparably higher and more complex than that of the animal and vegetable kingdoms, we still have a nature and we are better off when we live according to it instead of going against it.

Obviously there are different degrees of living with or going against our common human nature. I think that almost everyone would agree with me that the parents who killed their child would be going against our human nature in a most serious way; the same would be said about those who abused their child by beating or by seriously neglecting him. I would like to suggest that there are more subtle ways of going against our human nature, or at least of not really living in accord with it, and that this is particularly true in a culture that is fascinated by technology and "being modern." That fascination brought in the bottle and almost eliminated breastfeeding in America. Fortunately, there are an increasing number of people who recognize the wisdom of fostering the natural, and breastfeeding has made a comeback.

What we need is a lifestyle that incorporates a new respect for living in full accord with our human nature. For the present, this will also demand a new independence from the dictates of our contemporary culture. Such a lifestyle would support the close ties between a mother and her nursing child for as long as the child's needs kept him nursing. Since our present culture is not supportive of such a lifestyle, it is all the more important for every nursing mother to have loving support from her husband. When he is really with you, it matters little what others may think.

On the other hand, if a husband is indifferent or even hostile to the idea of breastfeeding and prolonged nursing, then other support may be in vain. Therefore it is extremely important that a nursing mother be a wife who communicates well with her husband. She should share not only her conclusions but likewise her reasons and the materials that she has found helpful and convincing. Many husbands will have open (or at least secret) admiration for a wife's ability to make an intelligent case for extended nursing.

Others will give their support if they see that the wife herself is really convinced and wants her husband's support regardless of how good a case she makes. What is important is that this be a shared decision so that the husband will be proud of his wife's willingness and desire to take care of their baby's needs in this way and so that the wife will find the support necessary to persevere in the face of cultural customs.

The strongest case for natural mothering and prolonged nursing is made by mothers who have raised one baby by our cultural standards and a later one according to the pattern of natural mothering. Repeatedly, those who changed their attitudes and allowed prolonged breastfeeding have found it to be a rewarding experience. It has been common for them to state that they wished they had nursed their previous children in a similar manner and that they feel that mothers are missing out on a valuable experience by weaning too early.

Thus far I have said almost nothing about prolonged breastfeeding and natural child spacing. However, I have mentioned previously that the women in our survey who followed closely the guidelines of natural mothering experienced an average of 14.6 months of amenorrhea: a few went up to and beyond two years. Obviously, this length of amenorrhea was possible only because of long-term nursing. There is no way of predicting the length of amenorrhea for any particular woman whether in the first year or the second year. The late return of fertility and menstruation will usually happen only in those women who let their babies continue to nurse beyond the first year and who have the body chemistry factors that are favorable to a later return.

References

1. Maria Montessori, *The Absorbent Mind* (New York: Dell, 1967) p. 88.
2. Eda LeShan, *How Do Your Children Grow?* (New York: David McKay, 1972) pp. 17-18.
3. — p. 18.
4. James L. Hymes, Jr., *The Child Under Six* (Englewood Cliffs: Prentice-Hall, 1961), p. 61.
5. Margaret Mead, "Working Mothers and Their Children," *Catholic World*, November 1970, p. 78.

12

Sex and the Lactating Mother

Certainly there are individual differences with regard to the sex drive, and one's sex drive may be influenced by several factors such as alcohol, fatigue, natural hormones including those during pregnancy and lactation, or artificial hormones (taking the Pill) and so forth.

Pregnancy and nursing may affect a woman's sexual drive. For those women who have no change or else find an increased desire, there is generally no problem. A few rather exceptional women find that lactation increases their sexual drive to such an extent that they experience erotic sensations. These women can accept these feelings as normal, not feel guilty or bad, and let these feelings subside naturally. Weaning the baby is not the answer. This situation is usually uncommon, but some women have been accused of nursing an older baby for their own sexual gratification.

On the other hand, women who find a reduced interest in sex while nursing may wonder if they are abnormal. One nursing mother told us she had a very strong desire to have sex with her husband during pregnancy (even prior to labor the urge was very strong), but immediately following childbirth she lost all interest in genital sex. Other women have written that while nursing they lost their desire for the genital embrace and wondered if something was wrong with them.

Some of these women have also read materials which give the impression that if you nurse, your love life will improve. That information can increase the worry and concern if you find that this is not your situation, but instead the exact opposite is true.

A decreased sex drive for the nursing mother appears to be very common. A home birth instructor who continues to have contact with nursing mothers after birth finds that almost all the breast-feeding mothers she talks to have lost their sexual drive. She claims the main reason is that the woman's body is constantly in touch with her baby and thus receives a sense of physical and emotional well-being in the motherly act of nursing. Women are cuddlers and caressers and the nursing mother derives a great deal of emotional satisfaction as her infant smiles, coos, touches her face, lips, chest and looks up into her face. These tender moments or emotional highs add to the emotional well-being of the mother.

On the other hand, hormones certainly cannot be ignored and probably play an important role in the changes which occur during these maternal times. For example, why do women have their sexual desires heightened during pregnancy but find it almost eliminated during nursing?

Dr. Michael Murray has pointed out that nursing mothers tend to have a reduced libido or a reduction in sexual desire, fantasy and need. He also notes that there is "a reduction of estrogen, the hormone which conditions and maintains vulvar tissues. Consequently, the nursing mother may continue to be over-sensitive and to become sore from genital contact and manipulation. Her breasts are also tender and sore."[1] However, breast soreness, if present, occurs briefly only in the early weeks.

There is a tremendous amount of time and energy spent in the care of a baby so fatigue can be a factor in reduced sexual feelings. I would hope fatigue would be a factor only occasionally since fatigue can be minimized if the mother is sleeping with her baby. A mother who takes time to take a nap, enjoy her baby and the nursing times together will be more refreshed than the mother who continually tries to get something done around the house or gets too involved with outside activities. I also believe that fatigue may decrease the milk supply, reduce the strength and occurrence of the let-down, and can bring an early return of menses.

Some remedies to physical changes that occur in a nursing mother's body are as follows:

Dry vagina. This can cause extreme pain or discomfort and can be relieved by an application of a water soluble lubricant such as KY jelly on the external lips of the vulva; KY jelly is not a contraceptive jelly. Vaseline is not water-soluble and is generally unsatisfactory as a vaginal lubricant. For a cost-free and always available lubricant, you might try your own saliva, applying it with white, unscented tissue paper. Another readily available lubricant is raw egg white, a substance also thought to aid sperm migration. Sometimes a topical estrogen cream is prescribed, but such creams have side effects. For example, the estrogen will be absorbed and may cause a mucus discharge, thus interfering with the observation of the normal signs of fertility.

Leaking breasts. Spraying of milk from the breasts during lovemaking is normal and should not be any concern to the man or the woman. If the woman chooses, she can apply direct pressure with her hands to each breast during a let-down. This prevents spraying and leaking and is used at other times by nursing mothers to avoid wet spots.

Sore breasts. This is common after childbirth and is usually eliminated by proper preparation of the nipples during the pregnancy. Some nursing mothers not only experience sore nipples but cracked and bleeding nipples as well. Obviously, at these times the breasts are temporarily untouchable, and great tenderness should be a main concern during lovemaking.

My advice based on personal experience and those of other nursing mothers is to administer treatment to the nipple area immediately once the tiniest amount of soreness is observed. Soreness, if it occurs, usually appears within the first few days of baby's frequent nursings, but it can occur later as well. I believe that coating the nipple with creams and lanolin only covers up the problem. Keeping the area dry is desirable, so change wet pads or wet bras. The quickest method of healing I found was the slow steady stream of warm air from a portable hair dryer. Apply the warm air to the breast often and especially after a feeding to dry the breast. Healing usually occurs quickly with these frequent applications.

Changes involving lovemaking. Your baby may cause a few scheduling changes. For example, if you and your husband are all ready for bed but your baby is awake and playful, be patient and enjoy your baby. The "family bed" is no real deterrent to marital intimacy because once your baby falls asleep, he can be placed elsewhere—or you can move yourselves. Because some babies tend to be very wide awake in the evening hours, sometimes parents find lovemaking more convenient in the early morning hours, lunch hour, the weekends, or baby's nap.

Even though the drive is absent, a wife can still engage in the marital embrace and enjoy lovemaking on the basis of loving and giving herself to her husband. The husband can appreciate his wife's feelings and not expect the same frequency of lovemaking nor the same strong response or the same type of foreplay from his wife since her sexual desires have changed.

Marriage will have various times of readjustments, and babies bring a new adjustment phase to marriage whether it's a first baby or a fifth baby. Parenthood brings new decisions, worries, concerns, times of happiness, and events which can influence love-making. Attitudes on parenting and children can surface which can affect lovemaking. The wife, for example, may talk constantly about the children when her husband is home instead of spending some time discussing his day.

Another example would be the feelings some women have with regard to child care. Her husband is so wrapped up with his job (or jobs), spends lots of time with some athletic team or hobby, or watching sport programs on weekends, that she feels child rearing is entirely on her shoulders. The wife no longer feels she is impor-tant and wishes her husband would spend some time with the chil-dren as well. Obviously, these feelings can happen whether a woman is nursing or not, and these feelings do affect lovemaking. A woman wants to feel loved and also that she is doing a good job of mothering. Secondly, she needs support from her husband. By his availability and his caring for her and the children, she likewise responds by loving and caring for him. I have often felt most loving toward my husband during these special caring times for me and at those times when he is relating to the baby or the older children. It is natural that a man's caring for his wife and children generates a loving wife.

Both partners can appreciate that nursing can be a positive time of togetherness for them. He can put his arm around her or they can share thoughts and plans for themselves and their children as she rocks and nurses the baby to sleep. Music, reading and prayer are other things a couple can share. Thus baby's nursing time does not mean "no husband" time. The wife may use non-nursing times to show affection--a greeting kiss at the door or snuggling up to read or watch TV.

Communication among caring partners helps during the read-justment periods, and that means talking about your feelings. A speech communication expert found that "married people talk to each other on an average of 27-1/2 minutes (that's minutes, not hours) a week."[2] The newspaper article pointed out how a good talk or conversation is extremely rare in today's world. Hopefully, those couples who give birth together and share in child-rearing and in natural family planning have already communicated in those areas and have found discussions related to their married life extremely valuable. Nursing is an excellent opportunity for such discussions. Shared parenting likewise can strengthen the mar-riage bond and family life.

Values, too, are important. If the two partners differ on values, the marriage will not be a good one even with lots of communication. If one partner does all the taking, and the other all the giving, communication does not help until the selfish partner begins to see he or she is self-centered.

Obviously, both partners must see that sex and marriage are so much more than genital. Their covenant for better and for worse covers the time of fertility and infertility as well as the times of a sexy-feeling wife and a not-so-sexy-feeling wife.

In conclusion, the husband can respond to his wife's changes in sexual desires with understanding, tenderness, affection and appreciation for the mother of his children. He can agree to have sex less and to be more of a helpmate with the baby or to do more activities with the older children.

He can also share with his wife in the emotional enjoyment of children by responding to his baby, playing with him, holding him, etc. She, in turn, can respond with affection and love for her husband, even during lovemaking when her bodily feelings do not seem to be there.

References

1. Michael Murray, "Sexual Problems in Nursing Mothers," *Medical Aspects of Human Sexuality*, October 1976, p. 75.
2. Beth Dunlop, "A Good, Deep Talk Isn't Cheap Anymore," *The Cincinnati Enquirer*, January 21, 1980, p. B-6.

13

Disappointments With Ecological Breastfeeding

Mothers who complain about ecological breastfeeding generally fall into two categories: 1) those who believe they followed the program but had an early return of menstruation, and 2) those who want another baby but are still infertile due to the breastfeeding. In the former situation, the mother feels the natural mothering program did not work for her, while in the latter situation the program works too well and a desired pregnancy seems impossible at the present time.

I. IT DOESN'T WORK

Our first concern will be those mothers who have an unexpected early return of their periods. I have collected five letters from mothers who informed me that the ecological breastfeeding program did not work for them. At the time I wrote each individually, but I would like to share excerpts from their letters and include a general response.

I must let you know that breastfeeding for child spacing didn't help in our case. At one month our baby would sleep from five to eight hours at night without nursing. We tried having her sleep with us but it just kept us awake, so we put her crib beside our bed. At ten weeks I got my first postpartum menstruation. Our baby never received a bottle, pacifier or solids until she was five months old.

I'm very much in favor of breastfeeding. I really think it's good for a baby to have the security of its mother. I am just letting you know that all

133

the rules for ecological breastfeeding were followed except for her sleeping with us.

From her birth I let Meagen set her own schedule, nursing as often and as long as she liked, and I never supplemented with water, juices or solids. By the time Meagen was three months old, she quit nursing through the night. When she was three and a half months old, I became pregnant. At that time I thought I was infertile due to complete breastfeeding.

If in fact, the early return of my fertility was due to not giving night feedings, then I wish you would overemphasize the necessity of night feedings in your newsletters. Although I still plan on complete breastfeeding with our next child, I also plan to chart from day one after leaving the hospital.

I'm writing because your method of natural child spacing happened to fail for me. I conceived when my daughter was about nine months old. I had no warning period whatsoever, I kept thinking I felt familiar symptoms of pregnancy, but could not believe it for quite awhile because I had such blind faith in your method. I breastfed right from the start and was still actively nursing her at this time — in fact she **still** nurses at least three or four times a day and still wakes up for an early morning nursing when sleeping [writer's emphasis]. I hardly ever left her with anyone for any length of time where she'd miss a nursing and have to take a bottle. So I can't understand how this happened.

I guess the main thing that made me a real believer was that it worked for me while I was nursing my son.

I belong to a breastfeeding support group and in the last year or so there were four other women that experienced the same thing. They became pregnant while nursing between four and ten months postpartum without a warning period. I think you are misleading a number of women like myself unless you make sure they know that it can and does happen.

I am now happy with my pregnancy and we are accepting it, feeling that it was meant to be and God wants us to have another!

With my first child I spotted at four months, resumed my periods at eight and a half months, and ovulated at 11 months postpartum despite very frequent nursing day and night. Why? Does the initial hospital schedule of four hours between feedings for the first couple of days have any effect? Otherwise, I have followed your guidelines completely.

I know that we have already agreed I am a special case, but I thought I'd pass this information along to you anyway. Increased suckling helps to stave off periods? Well, our newborn son is now two months old and I've just had my first period — the earliest, I think, I've ever had periods return. In addition to nursing the baby, I am also nursing our twenty-two-month-old and am collecting at least three ounces of milk a day for a sick baby! I'm disgusted with the malfunction of my body!

Following the rules. Anyone who has read this book or *The Art of Natural Family Planning* and anyone who has attended the natural family planning classes taught by the Couple to Couple League has learned that there are some cases where a pregnancy occurs before a first postpartum period and where menstruation returns earlier than expected.

We stress repeatedly **the importance of night feedings**. You cannot force night feedings, but expect an early return of fertility if the baby is not nursing during the night. One of the mothers wrote that four other acquaintances also conceived without a warning period. I have often discussed this situation with a friend who is the mother of nine children and who actively led La Leche League (LLL) meetings for over six years. With proper breastfeeding information which she gained from LLL, she achieved at least two years of amenorrhea with her latter babies. At the LLL meetings she met many mothers who claimed they conceived while totally nursing or without having had a period. Upon questioning, she found that not one of those mothers was nursing her baby at night. She stresses the importance of frequent nursings and that the night feedings are crucial for maintaining breastfeeding infertility. Frequent nursing doesn't mean you spend all day nursing the baby. Many times during the day a quick five- or ten-minute nursing is all the baby needs. An older baby receives a lot of milk in that short amount of time. Most of the longer nursings occur at naptime or during the night when the baby is tired.

Another mother mentioned she was actively nursing three to four times a day. I tell mothers that if their baby is down to five or six nursings a day, fertility can be expected to return soon if it hasn't already. Most mothers need lots of stimulation. As soon as the nursing pattern is reduced, fertility may begin to return.

Likewise, mothers who leave their babies can expect an early return of fertility. A rare quick trip to the grocery store when the baby is sleeping is one thing, but with natural mothering a mother soon learns how to take her baby with her to many different places. One mother said she rarely left the baby long enough that it would need a bottle. But apparently she was gone a few times for a long enough time that the baby did need a bottle.

In addition, some breastfeeding experts suggest that hospital restrictions on breastfeeding may interfere with breastfeeding infertility. These restrictions may come at a very critical time in the establishment of breastfeeding amenorrhea. Mothers should insist on unrestricted nursing from childbirth onward or choose a hospital that promotes mother-baby togetherness and unlimited nursing.

Disappointments With Ecological Breastfeeding   135

Body balance. It's possible that your height/weight ratio, your exercise pattern, and/or your diet may affect the duration of nursing infertility. To understand this, let's start with generally accepted principles for the non-pregnant, non-nursing woman.

Too little or too much body fat interferes with the normal menstrual-fertility cycle. Women who exercise excessively can develop either infertile cycles or runner's amenorrhea: in the first case they still have periods but such abnormal hormone patterns that they're infertile; in the second case they neither ovulate nor have periods. At the other end of the scale, obese women tend to have more menstrual-fertility problems than women of normal weight.

The generally accepted explanation for this is that the female sex hormones are fat soluble; if a woman has completely insufficient body fat, her sex hormones are processed by the liver and excreted before they accomplish their functions. If a woman has excessive fat, the hormones seem to be so absorbed by fat that once again they do not perform their intended functions in a timely fashion.

What about when you're nursing? Does your body fat ratio affect the duration of lactation amenorrhea? It's been determined that frequency of suckling is the primary ingredient, but as my husband and I have looked at the differences between different groups of ecologically breastfeeding mothers, we've begun to wonder if body balance might be a contributing factor. Thus we're starting to ask for some height-weight data on our revised breastfeeding survey. Our speculation runs along these lines: If you were obese before pregnancy and are still overweight, even considering the normal added weight of pregnancy, then we wonder if you might have either an early or a late return of fertility; if you were underweight before pregnancy and quickly lose your pregnancy gain, we wonder if you might have either an early or late return of fertility. Our guess is that where other factors are equal, women who are close to the norm for their height/weight ratio will come closer to the average duration of lactation amenorrhea than those who are far below or above the normal weight for their height and bone structure. That's strictly a guess; your recorded experience can add to the data we need. If you would like to participate in a periodic survey, write to CCL:BF Survey II, Box 111184, Cincinnati, OH 45211. Please mention this book, and we'll send you the survey.

Nutrition. Even if you're at the ideal height/weight ratio, you can have menstrual/fertility irregularities during times when you aren't either pregnant or nursing. For example, if you eliminate all

136

salt from your diet, you might experience an iodine deficiency unless you get iodine from another source such as regular seafood or kelp tablets. (That's why iodine is added to salt—iodized salt). Taking excessive vitamins may interfere with normal hormonal functions because both vitamins and your sex hormones are processed by the liver. Based on the role of nutrition on the menstrual/ fertility cycle when you're not nursing, it's possible that nutrition may also play a role in the duration of lactation amenorrhea while your're doing ecological breastfeeding.

Fatigue. Another factor that may interfere with breastfeeding infertility is fatigue. I am convinced that this is a time when a woman should be involved with her baby, husband and family and not be overly involved with the world and outside activities. It's a time to slow down and enjoy your baby. I'm not saying you should stop all involvement; however, outside activities should be minimal, and housework or activities should not cause excessive strain. Fatigue can hinder the milk supply and the let-down reflex. The mother who was nursing two babies plus expressing milk for another baby may have been overdoing it. One mother credited overwork to an early return. As she said, "I think my periods returned early from too much work during the canning season and I didn't get enough rest." When fatigue sets in, pre-menstrual feelings may develop. Your body is sending you signals to slow down and get more rest, so get adequate sleep during the night by not having late bedtime hours, and take a nap after lunch.

If fatigue is a problem, what can the nursing mother do to provide herself with more rest and relaxation? A bath with baby before a planned nap can relax both. Skin contact is at its best when mother and baby snuggle under the sheets after bathtime with minimal clothing. Another suggestion is to take time out to do something special for your baby. A walk can be just as much fun and refreshing for you as for the baby. A walking toddler soon runs well. Pick a large area of grass in the backyard or at a park or school and let him go. Let him walk the sidewalks, but bring him home (even under protest) if he keeps insisting on walking to the street. Crawling babies love the outdoors, the water trickling from the hose—even the sprinkler giving off a small amount of water. You can enjoy the baby's fun and the outdoors as well.

Take time out for the nursings. Sit down or lie down. Occasionally one might converse or read while nursing a baby to sleep; however an avid reader should put the book aside and interrelate with the baby during the nursing. The back and forth responses between mother and baby are important in the emotional development of the two.

Another suggestion is to eliminate coffee (or use a de-caf brand) in the mornings and before naptime for an easier sleep. Or at least limit yourself to one cup early in the morning with a good nutritious breakfast.

Reduced activities, a daily rest, and more relaxing times with baby (whether nursing times or "other" times) may eliminate the spotting, the pre-menstrual tensions or an early return of menstruation. On the other hand, a very small percentage of women may still experience an early return of menstruation regardless of following the above advice. In general, if your baby is sleeping through the night, if you have reduced your nursings, or if you are leaving the baby for a length of time, then begin natural family planning charting in anticipation of a probable early return of fertility.

II. IT WORKS TOO WELL

While many couples enjoy a long period of breastfeeding amenorrhea and infertility, it may become a source of frustration when the couple desires another baby. The nursing mother may try to eliminate a feeding or cut down on the nursing by doing other activities with the child. Occasionally this helps, but often in the natural mothering process the child is not ready to skip a feeding, and tears roll down his face. It becomes quite evident through his behavior that he still has a real need to nurse, and to try to skip that nursing when he is tired before naptime or bedtime is almost impossible. With child-led weaning these feedings are gradually dropped as there is no longer a need. But for many couples the frustration comes in waiting and waiting for a return to fertility. Some of these mothers are women who started having children later in life and see their reproductive years nearing an end.

A few couples will not be able to achieve pregnancy until after their child is completely weaned—even though they are having regular menstrual cycles and their chart shows the fertile signs and a beautiful postovulation thermal shift. Furthermore, the same woman may be unable to become pregnant while nursing one and conceive easily while nursing another. One friend was nursing an almost two-year-old and desired another baby. Her chart showed all the signs of fertility, but she could not achieve pregnancy. Dr. Konald Prem of the University of Minnesota Medical School, who helped us start the Couple to Couple League, told her she would get pregnant the first cycle after weaning. Eventually the child weaned and she did get pregnant the first cycle after weaning! I later ran into her when she was nursing her third child which she informed me she conceived while nursing her second baby. Thus in her case, history did not repeat itself.

Most couples can look to a return of menstruation as a sign of fertility if another baby is desired. But what happens if there is no return of menstruation? What are the feelings a couple is experiencing when they yearn for another baby but the mother is still experiencing amenorrhea? A mother wrote us about this particular problem which we shared with others in the Couple to Couple League (CCL) newsletter:

Our son will be three years old soon. Basically he nurses at nap, bedtimes, the odd time through the night, and on a bad day for comfort.

I have read the CCL manual and have been practicing natural family planning as much as I can. My menses has not yet resumed, so I began taking my temperature and observing any mucus and cervical signs— looking hopefully for ovulation in spite of having no period. However, my temperature remains fairly constant between 97.0 and 97.3. The cervix remains low, firm and closed; and to date there is no sign of fertile mucus.

All of this is unfortunately discouraging, as my husband and I wish to conceive again; I do hope for a return to fertility soon. I feel that any amount of sucking stimulation from my son is all that is necessary to suppress my ovulation. I'm sure I am on the long end of the scale for lactation amenorrhea. I do not wish to force weaning as I believe in allowing him to take the lead in his own development, but this does put me at odds— wanting to continue to meet my toddler's needs.

Child spacing of three years is what I had hoped for, but it may extend to four years. I had enjoyed natural mothering immensely until recently and this is, of course, due to wanting another child.

We received some excellent responses, and I would like to share them with you. They provide different insights to this particular problem.

I would like to share the experience of someone I know. The woman married and conceived in her early twenties. She weaned the baby at about one year due to cultural reasons. She could not conceive again until after six years when she conceived with the help of a fertility drug. She liked the idea of baby-led weaning, but when the sixteen-month-old was still nursing, she made the decision to wean so she could go back onto fertility drugs to achieve another pregnancy. She weaned her toddler (not too happily) and before she could begin the drugs, discovered she was pregnant. With this baby she was relaxed and didn't worry about hurrying the weaning. But she discovers she is pregnant when the baby is a year old and this pregnancy turns out to be twins. Four children under the age of four is a handful. The situation made for a strained marital situation and strained economic situation. How different her situation may have been if she had listened to her second baby's need to nurse a little longer. We never know what the future holds or what God has in store for us.

The three-year-old's mother has no guarantee that she will ever conceive again or that her second baby will not miscarry. If it turned out that this was your only child, would you regret having weaned him prematurely? Babies spaced four or even five years apart may not be what you planned, but consider that you are meeting the needs of your three-year-old who, after all, is only on loan from the Lord. If Jesus Himself had carried the baby to your front door and asked you to "take the best possible care of him," what would you do?

From a practical point of view, rejoice! You'll have the first child through college before the second child is there (not all bad). Take the best care you can of the child you have and trust in God for the children you hope for.

I always turn to your article first for support in my mothering style. My heart really went out to the mother who's nursing and wants to become pregnant. How discouraging to keep looking for fertility and discovering none. This difficult time can be depressing and makes it hard to enjoy the present time.

Take this special time in your son's life to enjoy him. Do other "mothering" activities such as trips to the park, reading, painting, etc. and you might notice your son's interest in nursing going down. If charting, please don't spend all your energy looking at the chart for long periods of time and fretting over it like I did.

Our four children were planned, but they never came in the exact month or even the year that they were longed for. I had to accept the fact that God was the Creator and it was difficult to accept, but the acceptance has caused my faith to grow in the long run.

I read an article in our La Leche League leader's newsletter some time ago about a mother with a nursing three-year-old. She also was unable to conceive until her doctor advised her to gain 10 pounds, which she did. She became pregnant within about three months after the weight gain without altering her nursing pattern.

I have a close friend who is very thin (5'6" and about 108 to 110 lbs). She breastfed two children, and menses did not return until each was completely weaned.

It is well-known that anorexic women do not menstruate. Perhaps some women are borderline and a few nursings a day are enough to suppress their cycles.

In regard to the woman who was writing regarding her lactation amenorrhea, I think this can raise a question: Can a couple be selfish in wanting more children? I'm not saying this couple is, but I do think we need to trust God's design and timing more. If her fertility has not returned but her youngest still needs to nurse, this couple may want to seriously consider that the "timing" may not be right for another pregnancy just yet. We planned our first child very deliberately but allowed God free reign with our second child. After 26 months of amenorrhea, I had four periods and conceived while charting laxly. If our baby had been born two weeks earlier or later, it would have been under extremely difficult circumstances. As it was, God's timing was exquisite.

It may be that more couples need to "listen" to the Lord more in guiding their family size and timing. It's food for thought and prayer anyway.

I experienced amenorrhea for two years and nine months while nursing my twin sons. I had anxiously awaited my period from about the time they turned two. I also thought a spacing of about three years would be nice. I did not encourage them to slow down the nursing. When my period returned, they were nursing just before bedtime and naptime. I did have a few months warning that fertility was returning by signs of mucus. I felt elated when I discovered that I was pregnant after only one cycle. I figured my plan of three years apart would only be altered by six months.

But then in my twelfth week of pregnancy I miscarried the baby. We were devastated. I felt like my whole life was just one big wait.

The next four months were miserable. My periods returned but they were erratic and ovulation was hard to pinpoint. Often my cycle was extra long and I would think I was pregnant again only to start a period on day 38 or 40. Finally I did become pregnant and delivered a healthy son when my older boys turned four. The child is now 20 months old.

Now that it's over, the time it took to have another child seemed short. However, at the time I became consumed with the thoughts of pregnancy. I felt as if my body had played a cruel trick on me. Here I was doing what I thought was best for my sons by breastfeeding them, and, in a way, was being punished for it.

My conclusion has been to reconcile myself to God's will for us as a family. He has a divine plan for us and by allowing nature to do her thing I am not interfering with that plan. God's ways are not our ways. He knows what is best for us and understands our destiny. We can never fully appreciate this with our limited knowledge and must therefore trust in Him when things are not going as we would like. This can be hard to accept as I well know, but I also know how fallible my decisions can be. To think about it honestly, I'm relieved to let this important decision about spacing and consequently the number of children up to God. He knows what He is doing. The challenge is for us to accept and adjust to it in a positive way.

Sometimes it is nice to receive a follow-up letter to hear how events turned out after a mother has written. The mother who was nursing the three-year-old and desired another child did write back. Here is what she had to say:

Thanks for your letter of support and encouragement earlier this year. Nature has taken its course and on this past weekend when my son turned three years old, I had my first postpartum menses.

We are now back to recording temperature and fertility signs after giving it up for several months. I reread *Breastfeeding and Natural Child Spacing* and a first postpartum menses of 39 months was mentioned. I thought I would give myself at least that long, and it has happened.

I had been prepared for eighteen months or two years of amenorrhea, but three years seemed impossible. However, I feel that it has proven best for our family. My son has always been a high need child and I'm sure he has needed all of this time alone. He is quite independent now and I feel he could accept my attention to a sibling. He would be about four years old when and if a new baby were to bless our family.

Our son still nurses at naptime and early evening before bedtime. I am sure the lack of night nursing is what finally allowed my hormonal system to return to normal cycles. I thought he was ready to wean, but he seemed to need his naptime nursing more than anything. Even when playing outside he'll stop play and tell me, "I need nappy. I need milky. Please, mommy." So we continue to enjoy this special time together. He is such a big boy in so many ways, but at this time he is still my baby who needs his mommy.

To think of nursing a toddler/child of this age would have been repulsive to me even when my first son was born; but having grown and evolved in this relationship together makes it so beautiful. Contact with La Leche League and the Couple to Couple League has given needed support and encouragement.

These disappointments over an early return of menstruation or over an extended amenorrhea are mentioned to help others who find themselves in a similar situation. Those who have an unexpected early return of menstruation may start charting for the return of fertility; if fertility returns, they can abstain according to the natural family planning rules in order to achieve the spacing they desire. Or they may choose to use natural family planning throughout their married lives and keep their family at its present size if they have a serious reason to do so. The couple who long for another baby can realize that God's plan for them at this time does not include another baby. In both situations, the woman is happier once she accepts her own natural pattern. The disappointment will hopefully only be temporary and she will go on from there, accepting the unexpected gracefully and finding support from others and maybe from this chapter.

14

Personal Experiences

There is ample research to show that the breastfeeding program described in these pages will normally be effective in child spacing, but most people are not going to review the sources I have quoted. Most of us learn best by example. Thus I have included the following experiences from friends who initially took an interest in the subject of natural child spacing and who helped me develop my ideas about natural mothering. Although these experiences occurred at a time when the primary emphasis was on child spacing through the total nutrition rule, their stories show that they were grateful for both the natural infertility and the nursing experience itself.

Their experiences likewise led me to write this book. For some reason, the physicians attending these women either did not or could not supply them with the information they needed at the time. They were most grateful for the information they received during our many conversations; and since this information was not available in book form, they encouraged me to put what we talked about into print.

MOTHER A

Mrs. A completely nursed her baby for five months before gradually introducing solids to her baby. Her first menstrual period occurred when her baby, her fifth child, was fourteen and one-half months of age.

At about three months following delivery, Mrs. A spotted, and the same thing occurred twenty-eight days later. Her obstetrician did not believe in the spacing benefit of breastfeeding and told her that her periods were trying to return. She and I were both puzzled by the spotting, as her baby was completely breastfed. Finally I asked her when she fed the baby during the night. She replied that her baby went to sleep early in the evening and awoke in the morning, quite content to go without an immediate feeding. We both felt that this long lapse in time may have been the cause of the spotting. She then took my suggestion to nurse her baby before retiring or else first thing in the morning. There were nights when her baby was too sleepy to nurse, and then there were nights when he demanded a night feeding. She also tried to increase his daytime feedings. No further signs of spotting or bleeding occurred until ten months later when she had her first regular period. Menstruation, in this case, was absent during the latter nine months (5 to 14 months postpartum) when the mother was giving her baby other foods. Her baby weaned himself at seventeen months of age.

Mrs. A could not convince her personal physician of the merit of breastfeeding in the area of family planning. As for her pediatrician, she was very reluctant to tell him that she was still nursing her baby. At the six-month checkup, she expressed her feelings on the matter, and expected that he would advise her to stop nursing. But to her surprise the doctor sat down, asked her some questions, and then admitted that he wished all mothers of his little patients would do exactly as she was doing.

Mr. and Mrs. A's previous babies had been born about a year apart. They were happy to have learned about natural spacing, for they wanted a larger family at a somewhat slower rate, and both liked the natural way of doing things.

MOTHER B

Mrs. B nursed her baby completely for five months. Soon after some solids were introduced, spotting occurred. The mother returned to complete breastfeeding and about two months later reintroduced solids because her baby wanted them. A regular period soon followed when her baby was eight months old. This was her fifth baby.

Mrs. B did not believe that breastfeeding would postpone another pregnancy. However, after reading the research and realizing that it is the sucking that is so important, she became convinced—and also was upset that her doctor hadn't told her about natural spacing with her first baby.

Mrs. B had several comments regarding the early return of menstruation after she introduced solids to her baby. First, she felt that the pacifier was her drawback. Since her baby used the pacifier regularly, he was never content to remain at the breast; her baby would not fall into a deep sleep at the breast like other babies. Maybe this additional pacifying-type nursing would have been all that was needed in order to hold back menstruation for a longer period of time after the baby began solids.

Secondly, she often used these solids to pacify the baby when all the baby wanted was her. If she was too busy to hold the baby, she found it more convenient to offer food to satisfy him. She came to regard this as a poor form of mothering. It also tended to limit the amount of nursing at the breast by filling up the baby with solids.

Mrs. B found several advantages in complete breastfeeding:

1. She was extremely happy to have learned about natural spacing and to have had peace of mind during the non-menstrual phase of breastfeeding.

2. With her previous babies, she had found carrying them during menstruation very uncomfortable because of pain in her legs. However, with her last baby this did not occur. Also, by the time most nursing mothers' periods resume, their babies are learning how to walk and do not need to be carried as much around the house. She feels that other mothers who are uncomfortable during menses would also benefit by nursing properly and experiencing a lengthy absence from menstruation.

3. Mrs. B strongly feels that the children are the ones who benefit immensely from the extra contact and attention that is part of natural mothering. She feels it is so much easier to do this when they are little than to try to make up for it in later years. Frequently when babies are born close together, the parents tend to treat the older baby as a grown child and fail to realize that they really have two babies in the house—both of whom need lots of babying and loving care.

4. And, lastly, she feels that if she had totally breastfed in the early months, she would have been able to nurse her other babies. Early introduction of bottles and solids was the cause of her nursing failures. When this was first written, her baby looked as if he would be an early weaner; at ten months of age he was nursing well only once during the day. The baby quickly lost interest in the breast once solids were introduced. Mrs. B plans to nurse until the baby weans himself; she is enjoying the relationship too much to stop, and she feels that babies should be nursed for about two years. Since in her locality it is extremely rare to hear of a mother still nursing a baby at even ten months of age, she doesn't plan to advertise the fact. "I don't feel I have to explain myself to others or

want to be in a position where I have to think up some reasons. I just want to and it's as simple as that."

MOTHER C

Mrs. C, a pharmacist from Australia, nursed her second child "completely" for seven months. Her periods returned when her baby was nine months old.

Since she wanted to quit nursing at three months for fear of becoming pregnant—a common belief that has unfortunately developed out of the cultural breastfeeding practices which normally do not provide a lengthy period of natural infertility— Mrs. C began to offer her baby some formula. Her pediatrician asked her why she wanted to stop nursing since her baby was allergic to other milks, and he then told her about proper breastfeeding in order to delay another pregnancy. He also told her that it would probably mean delaying solids for some time and then referred her to me.

As a pharmacist, this mother became extremely interested in the research material on the subject. She then remembered that her grandmother nursed all her children for two to three years and said it was the **only** way, and that her mother's advice was, "Be careful when you wean."

It is interesting to note that Mrs. C's baby went an unusual length of time between feedings for a breastfed baby. Her baby nursed every four to six hours during the day, whereas most babies nurse several times during that amount of time. From five weeks of age her baby slept through the night for twelve to thirteen hours. When the baby was four months old, she began to wake him to nurse before she went to bed because she felt that the long period without a feeding might force a return of menstruation. However, no bleeding occurred during those early months. Even though her baby did not nurse as frequently as mine or other babies, we figured that maybe our babies were spending about the same amount of time at the breast. Whereas my baby would nurse for about five to ten minutes at a feeding, her baby would nurse about twenty minutes at a feeding. Perhaps the time factor in a twenty-four-hour day wasn't as unequal as it at first appeared.

The attitudes of different doctors who saw this mother were interesting. The pediatrician saw no reason why this mother couldn't totally nurse her baby for nine months as long as the baby received some vitamin and iron drops. However, the obstetrician thought she was playing Vatican roulette and told her that she would be lucky if it worked. This doctor has told other nursing mothers that they should take other precautions or else he will be seeing them next year to deliver another baby. Mrs. C did not convince him; yet she relied on breastfeeding in spite of this doctor's opinions and in spite of her not wanting another pregnancy. Finally, at her last visit, the obstetrician said that he could see that it might work if a mother had a really aggressive baby—although this mother's baby was certainly not aggressive or very demanding at the breast.

Her general practitioner, on the other hand, was extremely interested in what she had to say and said he really learned something new. This doctor was very happy for her, said he would give the information to other interested patients, and also said he was especially pleased to see a healthy baby who was nursed so long on just mother's milk.

Mrs. C decided to let her baby continue nursing; plans for abrupt weaning gave way to understanding and enjoying the nursing relationship.

MOTHER D

Mrs. D nursed her third baby completely for seven and a half months. The baby was eleven months old when menstruation returned. The mother weaned the baby at sixteen months of age.

This mother introduced cereal a week before she learned about the spacing benefit of total breastfeeding. She called her pediatrician and he told her it would be all right to drop the cereal and to completely nurse the baby.

In Mrs. D's own words: "Most of all, the child spacing and 100 percent nursing were the greatest helps." She had nursed her other two babies, but she found that with this baby she had a very different and special relationship due simply to the complete breastfeeding. "I think 100 percent breastfeeding is the only way to start a baby out in this complex world of ours. For me it was the most wonderful experience of motherhood I have ever had."

AUTHOR'S EXPERIENCE

I wish I could say that someone had given me adequate instruction about breastfeeding with our first child, but the fact is that like most mothers I was really quite unknowledgeable about it. As a result, our first baby was not totally breastfed. I used bottles occasionally and began solids at five months. My first period occurred at three months due to early weaning. I thought at the time that this was a natural occurrence since my obstetrician told me I would have a period within three months following delivery regardless of how I fed the baby. Little did I realize until later how "un-natural" this occurrence was if you take nature as your norm. Weaning was completed at 10 months; in fact during the last two months of nursing I was only able to provide milk at one breast. The use of bottles interfered with lactation; there were times when John encouraged me to nurse instead of relying more and more on the use of bottles.

In those days we were also doing things that are not advocated in this book. John and I were very much a part of our culture. In parenting our first child, we used pacifiers regularly as well as bottles for water and juice. We thought nothing of leaving our first baby in the care of others, and John had somehow gotten the idea that it was beneficial for her to have different sitters. We both felt very strongly that she should have her separate bed and bedroom, and I would never nurse lying down for fear of smothering her. Nursing at night was a chore since I sat up, often cold and tired. In addition, I was also a part-time working mother. Before graduation at a major university, my classmates and I were told by our professional staff that we should continue to work when we had children, that we owed it to society since the state had put so much money into our education.

I had planned on permanently leaving my job after the birth of our first child, but my boss made a special plea for my return and I resumed work two afternoons a week. Even then I could never understand how my classmates could leave their babies all day; a half-day for me seemed long enough. But now if history could repeat itself, I would have stayed home where I belonged. So you can see that we have changed considerably in our growth as parents.

We did have a two-year spacing between our first two children, but that was due to two miscarriages in between. One of the miscarriages occurred when nursing. My concern was if the nursing caused the miscarriage, but I was informed by the local medical doctors I spoke with and also by La Leche League International that nursing is not a factor in a miscarriage.

After our second baby was born, I picked up considerably more information about total breastfeeding. As a result, I completely nursed a baby for the first time. I also started sleeping with the baby for naps and night nursings, a practice I would not consider with our first child. My periods started at twelve months post-partum. While nursing this baby, I was also encouraged by the fact that I knew two mothers who completely nursed their babies while I was doing so. One of the mothers was Mrs. A, mentioned previously; the other mother nursed completely for nine months, and menstruation returned when her baby was about eighteen months old. She was still nursing and giving night feedings at this age. Menstruation for all three of us did not resume until our babies were twelve to eighteen months old.

When I informed our pediatrician of my plans, he was most interested, since he admitted not knowing anything about it. During our visits he never once made a reference to solids or juices. When the baby rejected the vitamin drops, he said that they were not that important but that I should make sure my diet was good. He checked her iron before and again after she reached six months and found everything satisfactory. Most of all, he was pleased with her health and good disposition.

I admired this particular doctor—not only for his medical knowledge and interest in breastfeeding—but for a special reason: he respected my right to decide when I should offer my baby something besides breast milk. I hinted, and even asked for his opinion as to when I should begin solids. He never answered that question. Neither he nor my husband would offer an opinion, other than letting me know I was free to go as long as I desired and as long as the baby continued to thrive on breast milk. The decision was thus entirely mine. At eight months, our baby showed her first tooth, so I took this eruption to mean a time for weaning. At least it became the answer to my question, "How long?" However, if the tooth had erupted at four or six months of age, I would have ignored this sign; if the baby were unhappy and needed the solids, I would have begun solids earlier. The introduction of solids at such a late date in no way detracted from her health or disposition. Only her mother knew when people commented how well she must eat or asked if she was that good all the time.

Our girl thus became familiar with non-milk foods and took a sip occasionally from a cup. I continued to offer the breast so that she was still receiving most of her liquid diet from me. At age eighteen months she came down with a cold, and I took advantage of the opportunity to wean her. That type of weaning is inconsistent with what I recommend in this book, and I would do it differently today.

Our third baby was born when our second was twenty-four months old. She was also nursed completely for eight months, at which time she began taking solids. Menstruation returned at ten and a half months—exactly fourteen days after she had a slight illness. During the illness she had a good disposition but a large decrease in appetite for any food including breast milk. This reduction in the amount of suckling for a two-day period caused, I feel, a premature return of menstruation. At about this time we came across a natural family planning article by Dr. Konald Prem from the University of Minnesota Medical School. Little did we know then that this doctor later would be instrumental in helping us start the Couple to Couple League so we could share information about natural family planning and ecological breastfeeding with other couples.

Our fourth and fifth children were nursed completely according to the natural mothering program. I am convinced from my reading of the literature and from our parenting experiences that natural mothering via breastfeeding provides the best start for baby as well as a rich emotional development for both mother and baby. The frequent, unrestricted nursing associated with natural mothering usually provides a natural spacing of births by suppressing ovulation for a full year or more.

You will notice that the emphasis in these personal accounts is primarily on total breastfeeding. In the 1960s total breastfeeding was the only rule given if you wanted to delay fertility. These accounts were from friends in those days who were learning about "total breastfeeding" and applying it in their personal lives. I would like to stress, however, that total breastfeeding is only one piece of the "natural infertility" pie. While this aspect of breastfeeding is important, the other practices advocated in this book are of equal importance in maintaining postpartum infertility. In my discussions with other interested mothers, it soon became apparent that other factors contributed to child spacing. During the parenting of our second and third children, many of these natural mothering concepts were discovered, and the "natural mothering" or "ecological" breastfeeding program was developed. In the late sixties and early seventies, "ecology" was almost like a new religion; it was constantly in the news media with regard to pollution and population. It seemed appropriate at that time to coin the term "ecological breastfeeding" to stress nature's way and to set it apart from the cultural nursing of most American mothers. Thus the "total breastfeeding" rule soon became just one part of the complete "ecological breastfeeding" program.

15

The Mail Box

NATURAL CHILD SPACING

Mothers who have written me after reading the first version of this book have three themes running through their letters: 1) they lack support from doctors and relatives; 2) they are deeply appreciative for the information and support given by La Leche League; 3) they experienced longer amenorrhea by following the natural plan for mothering.

These mothers wrote from the United States, Canada, Australia, and New Zealand. Here are some excerpts from a few letters expressing their thoughts and experiences on the subject of natural spacing and mothering. I am including them because many mothers find support in knowing about the experiences of others.

"God didn't mean for women to become 'baby-factories,' giving birth to a new child every year. In order that our bodies could recuperate from childbirth and build-up strength for a next pregnancy, He planned that breastfeeding would render us infertile for one to two years. Why should we bother with foams, artificial devices or the pill? God's plan is so much nicer!"

"You may also wonder if I am of a faith that does not condone birth control means. No, I am not, and I have in fact taken the pill for a year and a half between my two children. My boys are over three years apart, as I remained sterile for nearly a year after those pills. So I've found breastfeeding a lovely blessing in every way, and the infertility is only a convenient side effect. We've decided on a third child at the earliest possible date—considering the breastfeeding situation, of course."

"I'd just like to say I feel certain breastfeeding has a very definite effect on child spacing. With my other bottle-fed children I conceived again at eight months after delivery despite other contraceptives. So far it has been fifteen months since the last baby was born. No period yet."

"I first read your book when Lynda had nearly weaned herself. It certainly makes sense, and I am looking forward to having another baby. I only wish I had known more when Lynda was a baby because contraception can be such a worry. I would **never** go on the pill again."

"Our number one baby was twenty months old when number two was born. Our number two was thirty-four months old when number three was born. I nursed numbers one and two for about one year together. A lot of people have questioned me—"Is that all you're doing?" I tell them I have faith. It has worked for us and I really believe in it."

"My husband and I are very pleased with this most natural means of spacing children. It is especially great these hectic months after birth when tension over effectiveness of other methods and adjustments to a new baby can put a strain on a marriage. We feel this way is best for our family in every way and are overjoyed it works so well."

"Our fifteen-month-old is still nursing three or four times a day. For a while it seemed he wasn't too interested, except early in the morning. I haven't had a period yet. The other day someone was complaining of cramps and discomfort with her period and I mentioned that since my first baby I have never had all that cramping and pain with my periods. Then I said, 'But come to think of it, I've had so few periods.' And my friend said, 'You know, you are the truly liberated woman!' How true! So far I have had eleven periods in over eight years. This is with three babies."

"I just finished reading your book. Very informative! I just wish I could have read it twenty years ago! Our little girl wakes at night to be nursed and sometimes nurses often at night. We have a kingsize bed so it really doesn't bother our sleep. We have relied totally on nursing for preventing a new pregnancy. It is the most enjoyable method of spacing babies. I just regret all the years that were completely safe or could have been and we didn't know it."

152

"As a Protestant, it had never been presented to my husband and me as a logical way to have a family. Our sweet little one is nine days old, and she will be the first one not to have a soother. Many of my acquaintances are put right on the IUD after their first baby, and I think it's a shame when God intended His way of spacing little ones."

"We now know why breastfeeding spaces babies—the baby is always in our bed to nurse at night!"

"This is the only method of child spacing that appeals to my husband and me in every possible way. Myself, I look for simpler answers—ones that women in nontechnological societies might discover—and in breastfeeding I found it."

"Perhaps the future of the family is at stake in this generation, but I have faith in God that perhaps some of the turmoil the world is going through will make us return to the warmth and love, the heartaches and the pride that can come from close family unity. Developing as human beings is the only thing that can have meaning in a world that so often labels us as numbers. Breastfeeding and natural family planning can give us direction as families by turning us toward humanness."

"When my doctor spoke to me in the hospital, he was pleased I was going to nurse and asked that I not give solids until at least a month. I said: 'Great, I wasn't intending to introduce them for four months or more.' He said: 'I fully approve, but I think you had better begin with some cereal or other iron food around four months or have a blood check.' That's a pediatrician I like! He also said he usually has to fight his mothers and gives in at one month for solids. Nursing Lisa has been a beautiful experience. She is a wonderful, contented baby. Her weight gain has been well above normal and her iron level measured at six months was fine. She gave up that 2:00 a.m. feed very early at about six weeks. At three months she gave up the 10:00 p.m. feed, so I had that long stretch without nursing at night again. I went back to night feedings but she gave up one of her daytime feedings so I was still on four feeds a day. I spasmodically fed her at night but it was obvious she did not want it, so I finally gave up and she seemed happier. At six months she went to three feeds a day with four every now and then. I began solids around five and a half months with small pieces of banana and gradually introduced other foods. Lisa was really ready for solids and took to them greedily. I always nursed her before solids. Now she eats three meals a day and I cut out her midday nursing. However, she has been sick, and the last three nights with high fever she has gone back to nursing as nothing else makes her happy. One would expect a return of periods and/or ovulation with such a decrease in nursing, but apparently I must be able to keep the levels of 'inhibitory hormone' high enough to prevent ovulation."

"My second child is now seven and a half months old. I haven't had a period yet. I totally breastfed him until six and a half months when he wanted food from my plate. I learned from experience that I must be careful about introducing solids. My baby nurses twice at night and for long periods of time."

"Our fourth baby was born at home because we wanted no interference with hospital schedules. Because of this we nursed almost continually from a few minutes after birth until she was twenty-five hours old. The only times she wasn't at breast were when I was otherwise occupied—i.e., changing pads. This was beautiful for both of us. My milk was in at sixteen hours and she passed all the black stool by two days of age. She (six and a half months old) is now having one meal of solids per day. This is mainly meat, a few ounces of our regular table food. She has never slept in a bed other than ours since birth. She nurses on and off during the night, but I really don't know how often. I sleep nude from the waist up, so does the baby, in order to allow more skin contact. Consequently she eats whenever she likes. We use no other form of birth control so I imagine our next baby will come along in two years. My husband and I are both enjoying this fourth baby. It's my husband's idea to have her sleep with us. He feels she will benefit greatly by the close cuddling she gets at night. With three other children to care for, he feels the baby may not get enough holding and loving during the day. Therefore, he wants to ensure her getting her share of me at night."

"It has been my observation in three years of talking to nursing mothers, that night feedings are a critical factor in extending the time of postpartum amenorrhea, and that taking the baby to bed with you is a critical factor in extending night feedings. May I make a suggestion? It helps to stop thinking in terms of the bedroom and consider a sleeping room, with safe, low mattresses where the baby always sleeps. Then supplement this with a nearby, comfortable area to which the husband and wife may

154

retire if they wish privacy. Many of the 'overwhelming problems' of breastfeeding are really problems of logistics—confining floor plans, furniture, clothes, etc., which dictate a lifestyle that conflicts with breastfeeding."

"This was the first baby totally breastfed for six months, and also a true baby-led weaning. The assurance I got from my husband was what I needed. He really acted as a buffer against the relatives and friends. My doctor was a tremendous help by his positive attitude. It also helped to be able to quote his remarks to the relatives. The baby nursed very infrequently, but gained three pounds every month for the first six months except one month he gained four pounds. I am currently nursing our seventeen- month-old baby without a return of my periods."

"Baby sucked her fingers a lot the first three months when I tried halfheartedly to follow a schedule. She stopped when I really relaxed and fed her as often and as long as she needed."

"I believe not only in lying down while nursing but also in sleeping with one's children. My son nursed on and off through all of his nights. He is twenty-two months old and I have not yet had a period. Sleeping with one's children is so easy, so natural, so safe, so warm and loving."

MOTHER-BABY TOGETHERNESS

Practicing mother-baby togetherness can be difficult in a society where early separation is done so frequently among most mothers. This section of the mail box is devoted to mothers and fathers who would like to keep their baby with them; they will find support from others who have dared to be different.

"Last summer when I was seven months pregnant, my father died suddenly of a heart attack, leaving me to run the family retail business with my younger brother. I decided I had to carry on the business he had worked so hard to establish. I was determined to take the baby to work with me. He slept contently most of the time, and when he needed to nurse, I took him into an adjoining room where we had privacy. As time went on people began to remark on how placid and friendly he was. As for me, I never felt or looked better in my life. I was bursting with energy. So much for all the stories that breastfeeding is tiring and takes so much out of you."

"Here on the Air Force base, when a woman is pregnant, one of her priorities is finding a babysitter. We are considered strange because our baby is always with us. Our most difficult situations have been military functions. We carry the baby and ignore the odd glances. We like to make our ideas known in a gentle way when talking to people, but are careful not to be pushy or obnoxious. We have attended two formal military functions with the baby. In those cases we brought along a young twelve-year-old friend who cared for him in the lobby of the officers' club. I slipped away from time to time. We have found that our style of parenting requires more creativity, but obstacles can usually be overcome. Sometimes an activity must be given up temporarily."

"I have five breastfed children, but it wasn't always easy. With the first one I felt very tied down with breastfeeding. I made sure she would take a bottle so I could get out and get away once in awhile. When I look back now, the problem was that I wasn't comfortable nursing around others. I have overcome this. I have taken my nursing babies to concerts and picnics...even to the Democratic County Convention. Going on nature hikes is easy with a nursing baby. I've nursed baby at church by covering the baby with a blanket.

Our last three babies slept with us for two years. Even though I'm 38 now and have a five-month-old, I've never felt tired like I did with our first one who slept in a crib in a separate room. It's also nice to nurse the baby and read to a pre-schooler at the same time. The truth has set me free."

"I must admit there are some things I will not do again. The most prominent one is never leaving a baby with a sitter. I was pressured by our society rather than following my own instinct here. I also really resisted sleeping with my baby. But because of my illness and the baby's illness, we came to family sleeping and I discovered how wonderful it could be! I certainly got more sleep, and she seemed to sleep better with us than in her own room."

"I believe our daughter is above average in intelligence. I realize I may not be objective, but I hear the same thing from many other people who have come in contact with her. She is very friendly and outgoing and likes to play with other children or adults. This is in

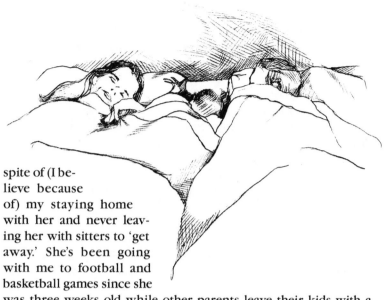

spite of (I believe because of) my staying home with her and never leaving her with sitters to 'get away.' She's been going with me to football and basketball games since she was three weeks old while other parents leave their kids with a sitter."

"Joshua has been a real joy. He's been to the mountains, the Gulf of Mexico, flown in an airplane, and helped me drive the combine at age six weeks. Truly a portable, happy, easy-to-care- for baby. I'll never go back to cribs and bottles."

"In 1980, my husband and I went to Italy and France with our four-year-old daughter and nine-month-old son. Many tour groups do not allow young children on their tours, so we did a lot of research about where we wanted to go and what we wanted to do and went on our own. We had planned this trip as far back as when I was pregnant with Paul, and when our plan to travel became known to friends and family, it was met with mixed reactions. Some thought it was a neat idea to take our kids, and some thought we were crazy. We didn't think it would be a burden since I nursed Paul.

Since we had plenty of time to plan, we figured out how many disposable diapers to take, how much clothing would be needed, and what we would carry around on a daily basis in a backpack. We purchased a Gerry carrier so I could comfortably carry Paul and still have my hands free. The airlines arranged for us to have a 'sky cradle' so Paul could have a place to sleep during our transatlantic flight.

We had a wonderful time and having the children along proved to be a real blessing. Everywhere we went, the people went out of their way to make sure we had what we needed and that we got good seats on the trains and local transportation. Everyone stopped to smile at our family, to hug the kids, and to make conversation.

Whenever necessary, I was able to nurse Paul, and I never had to worry about formulas or local food that might make him sick. It really was no problem for us. Nursing Paul provided an easy way for us to travel. All it took was planning and organization to make a successful trip.

Now we have three children (ages 8, 4, and 2) and we are planning to go to Italy this summer. Even though I won't be nursing a child on this trip, it is nice to know that if I were, it would not keep me from traveling."

"First I want to thank you for the positive effect you've had on my mothering skills. I nursed my first baby for four and one-half months and then quit because of the 'inconvenience'. I nursed my second baby for twenty-two months because it was so very convenient. The only thing that changed was my attitude and finding a supportive group of friends.

When our second baby was seven or eight months old, we had our annual family reunion at a campground. My two sisters had babies one month younger than mine and watching them at this camp-out made me thankful I was nursing. They were constantly warming up bottles by heating water on the Coleman stove (no fast procedure) and worrying about saving opened bottles in the ice chest and wondering how long they would keep safely. Then once a day my two sisters worked together washing and sterilizing bottles and nipples, and again needing to heat water on the Coleman stove. At night, one sister warmed a bottle and put it under her sweatshirt so she could keep it warm for her baby's nightfeeding. She didn't want to heat a bottle at 1:00 a.m. I won't mention the process involved in fixing their cereals and baby food, but it too was time consuming.

Compare their methods of feeding to my method which was breastfeeding. All I needed to do when my baby was hungry was to find a place to sit. Night feedings were even easier. My husband and I zipped our two sleeping bags together and there was room for the three of us. When the baby whimpered, he was immediately satisfied and we were both back to sleep within minutes.

When our second child was a year old, we drove ten hours from Michigan to Iowa. I could nurse him without unbuckling his car seat. I'd have to take my seat belt off though. Again nursing was very convenient. We usually would stop the car to nurse because it was more comfortable for me to hold him in my arms. And our three-year-old appreciated the nursing breaks as he got to get out of the car and play with dad. Also my periods resumed at 20 months postpartum. I enjoyed not having periods for that long."

"My insistence on staying with my ten-months-old daughter landed us an unplanned appearance in Paramount Pictures' *The Hunter,* Steve McQueen's last film! It was filmed in the Chicago area in the fall of 1980. Some of my family members are models and had landed parts as extras for the three weeks of filming in Chicago. After the Chicago filming, the set moved to some rural areas near Kankakee, where we live. When my mom (who was in the filming) heard that they were coming down, she suggested that they call me to help find people for the stand-in parts.

The agent asked me to come and take a part. 'No,' I said, 'I have a ten-month-old nursing baby. 'It's only for a half day,' he responded. I knew this meant seven or eight hours to them. 'That's too long to leave her', I said as my heart sank. He told me it would be O.K. to come and watch, and bring her if she's quiet.

As we observed the filming at the Kankakee Airport, the assistant director got an idea. Although he did not know me at all, he picked me and my baby from the observing crowd and told us to be in the next scene.

We rehearsed a few times, and discovered we would be in a scene **with** Steve McQueen. There were four of us and the pilot in the small plane. I sat across from Steve McQueen, knee-to-knee, with Susie on my lap. He mentioned how good she was and talked about his own daughter. Throughout the rehearsals, the shuttles, the practicing getting off and back on the plane, and being passed around, Susie was an angel.

Knowing that many hours of taped scenes are always cut from the final film, I was surprised to see myself and Susie in the premiere showing ten months later. A still shot of our scene with McQueen holding Susie returns again at the very last background for the credits at the end of the film.

Of all the stand-ins available, our mother-baby togetherness was the key to this once-in-a-lifetime experience for us. A few months after the filming, we received in the mail a large laminated wall plaque with a photo of our scene. It is personally inscribed 'To Coleen and Susie, from a fan...Steve McQueen.' The following October, McQueen died of cancer. It was truly a privilege to have met this man, and experienced some of his kindness toward children."

"I have followed mother-baby closeness with both Owen and

Paul and I believe that it was a big help to their development and to their sense of security. I can see my children developing into loving people who value people over things—that is the way we have treated them.

It seems to me that those parents who reject natural mothering may be saying that there is only so much giving that can be expected and 'I have my own life to live. This baby isn't going to change everything about my life!' Although this seems very selfish to me, many mothers feel entirely justified in this belief.

Then there are those mothers who believe the best thing for their babies is to be taught to be a 'good baby' whereas I believe my babies will teach me to be a good mother. I think these mothers are sincere in trying to do what is best, although from my perspective that seems to be what is most convenient. Eventually the baby will sleep through the night and will be comfortable with lengthening separations from mom.

If we are called to see Christ in everyone, then we should certainly see the baby Jesus in our babies. I often ask myself how would the Blessed Mother handle this or that problem. Thanks for bringing this part of natural family planning to so many mothers."

"My husband and I had it all planned. We would have a baby in a hospital and I would nurse for several months. The baby would sleep all night by three months of age and we would have a regular sitter so we could go out. Little did we know how parenthood would change us. We listened to each other and grew. Decisions were often painful and difficult to make.

Adam was born to us in an alternative birthing center. The three of us were never separated and we returned home the same day he was born. We needed our baby near us and we often brought him to bed with us for those night nursings. At age two weeks he developed colic and the family bed became reality as a matter of survival.

Adam did not do well without me. He needed me intensely and I was unable to leave him even for an hour. He nursed about every 1 1/2 to 2 hours around the clock for ten months. I knew from my LLL group that I was meeting the needs of my child and yet I often felt inadequate. It seemed other mothers had extra time for showers, reading and cooking. Adam's naps were often only twenty minutes long. This led to many feelings of frustration and anger. And yet, as we watched Adam grow, we knew we were making right decisions even though our family and friends often disagreed with us.

Adam went everywhere with us. He attended weddings, parties, meetings, and peace rallies. Now at fifteen months he is very active, happy and friendly. He still goes almost everywhere with us but once in awhile we leave him with friends for a couple of hours to take in a movie. He seems secure with this and does just fine. As for natural mothering, we would do it all over again. It does take support of like-minded friends and a dedicated spirit."

"First, I'd like to give you an idea of my background. I worked in a technical career involving computers and mathematics for about seven years prior to the birth of my first child two years ago. I was convinced of the importance of a child being raised at home by a parent, yet I had a strong need to maintain my career and stay technically-oriented. I decided to fulfill both needs by staying home with my daughter during the day and getting my doctorate on a part-time basis (two evenings a week) while my husband watched the baby. Clare was never without one parent until we went out to dinner when she was seven months old and we left her with a sitter.

From seven to seventeen months, she was left with a sitter no more than three or four times. I decided to attend a technical seminar for three days when Clare was seventeen months old. This meant I was away from her from seven to nine hours per day. I wasn't that worried about leaving her since my parents were coming down to watch her and she was able to go that long without nursing. It was while I attended this seminar that I found out the primary benefit of mother-baby togetherness.

The first morning of the seminar I nursed Clare in bed as usual. After she finished she did her typical hugging and caressing me. All I could think of was how hard it would be to leave her. Clare got along great with my parents and I had an enjoyable time at the seminar, so much so that visions of going back to work full-time danced in my head. However, what really made me reconsider was how Clare treated me after the seminar was over. She still nursed as often as usual but the hugging and caressing had stopped. Not only that but at times she even preferred to play with my mother rather than with me. I thought what it would be like to have Clare be more responsive to a total stranger (i.e. a babysitter I'd have hired) rather than her own mother. Fortunately, the three-day seminar did not totally shatter our relationship. After spending an entire day with Clare, the loving relationship continued where it left off.

I enjoy being at home and watching my child grow both physically and mentally before my eyes. I feel more in tune with my child's needs and can raise her the way I want instead of being at the mercy of her caretaker. I'm not worried about her safety or possible abuse because she is always with us or is cared for occasionally by a person whom we trust.

The most difficult aspect of mother-baby togetherness involves taking our baby along to some events in which she is not really welcome. It's hard to find friends that share the same values that you do. The first few times I left Clare with her father or sitter proved to be pretty traumatic for her and me alike. I don't know who missed whom more. Even now I have a tendency to put off getting a sitter for a night out because there is still some separation anxiety for both of us.

Sometimes I wonder whether we're doing the right things for our daughter. She tends to be more shy than other children who are with others on a regular basis. Having to cope with criticism from the grandparents who feel our daughter should be weaned or that we pay too much attention to her makes things difficult on occasion. Fortunately, the Couple to Couple conference in Baltimore helped reinforce that we are doing the best possible thing for our daughter."

"We have one daughter who is two and one-half years old and who is still nursing. She has gone everywhere with us since she's been born and really it has been no problem. In fact we are so at ease knowing that she is with us and having her needs met by us that the word babysitter is an obsolete word in our household.

The first public place we took Mary was to church. At first I was not comfortable nursing in public so I asked our priests to please put a chair in the church's bathroom. (I asked them if they thought they would enjoy nursing a baby on a toilet seat.) They gladly obliged. Later as I became more relaxed and more adept at discreetly nursing, I stayed in church and nursed.

Other outings included eating at restaurants. We would bring Mary along and set her in her infant seat. If she needed to be fed, I simply put a receiving blanket over my shoulder and proceeded to nurse her. I do remember the first time I nursed her at a restaurant. I was not real good at getting her started while being discreet about it at the same time. I simply excused myself, took her to the restroom and got her started there. Once she was on, I returned to the table and we both enjoyed our meals. That is a great advantage of breastfeeding—you have one hand free to feed yourself if your little one is hungry at meal time too.

Once while we were at a restaurant I noticed another mother nursing her baby. She had situated herself in an out of the way corner of the restaurant. She had a much more confortable spot to nurse in than I did. Our table was out in the middle of the floor. I felt very conspicuous. That situation taught me a lesson. In the future when we dined out, my husband always asked the hostess to put us in a corner or at least along a wall if possible.

My husband, Mary and I have also gone together to see movies at our local theater. We have always gone to the 9:15 p.m. show. That way we knew she would be tired and ready to nurse herself to sleep.

Ours is a large family so we have had the opportunity to take Mary to several weddings and wedding receptions. During the church service we usually sit towards the rear so an exit is easy if necessary. This is very important now that she has entered the trying two age. Oftentimes church services are very difficult because they don't offer too much excitement for a two-year-old. We simply recognize this fact and remain versatile. At the reception we come prepared with an appropriate size chair for her to sit in and her own spoon and fork. She has always loved all the excitement that goes along with wedding receptions. When it is obvious that she is tired, we either leave or put her in her portable buggy. Even with all the noise going on around her, she has never had any problem falling asleep.

So as you can see we really have fun taking Mary along with us. All that is necessary is a little advance planning so that we bring everything along that will make our outing comfortable for her."

"Jennifer went everywhere with us. The fact that I had to work part-time as a secretary-bookkeeper for the school district did not hamper our mothering style in the least. Through the 'divine' suggestion of the district administrator, we worked out a unique working relationship. Our baby was a 'colicky' baby; she nursed frequently and sucked endlessly. My husband's union contract was ending with talks of a strike, so I knew I had to keep working. While I was on my postnatal leave, the administrator brought my work to my home. I stretched my vacation days to reduce my work days. When that ended, Jenny was still colicky and I was frazzled by the rush-rush pace. My boss then suggested coming in on Saturdays with baby, and my husband could care for her while I worked.

So Saturday was an excursion to school. We made ourselves at home in the administrator's office and between feedings I did the district's bookkeeping. Jenny had many hours of back packing and crawling tours of the school classrooms. She was rocked to sleep in the 'Executive' chair. The Home Ec. room was our kitchen for lunch. An impossible situation to combine work with mothering was solved for a short duration. It was the first in this school district. I am most thankful to the administrator and his working suggestion of bringing the baby!"

"Emily would not take a pacifier or any bottle; she would only nurse. Therefore, she went everywhere with us. This was fine with my husband and me, and our baby was happy and content. When she was three months old, we had a chance to go to Puerto Rico. Children were not allowed on the trip, but we were going to try and take Emily anyway. When we arrived at the hotel, the man in charge of all the arrangements asked me if I had received the letter explaining 'no children.' I told him our baby came with us because she was totally breastfed. He seemed to be concerned about all the 'needs' the baby would need. I said we do not need a baby bed, food, or sterilized bottles. We were not allowed in the casinos nor allowed to see a stage show because no children were allowed. One evening when everyone else went to a show, we were given our dinner on the house. The room was private with candle-light. We had two guests: a little girl and her babysitter. The little girl belonged to the man in charge! He had brought his own daughter along on the trip.

Another time we took her on a couples' retreat for the weekend. She slept with us and never cried during the night because of the nursing. I felt good about taking her because her needs were being met."

"Our biggest challenge was the acceptance from others of our baby being with us. A cross-country ski group attracted us because of their encouragement of family activities. At three months of age, Dusty went to Cragun's in Brainerd, Minnesota, for a skiing escapade. Many club members remarked on how good he was for the six-hour bus trip there, the skiing itself, and the return bus trip. It is not hard when kids learn to be with mom and dad in all their activities. Just last week, we again trekked to Brainerd. This time Dusty was on skis and his eight-month-old sister was in a Gerry carrier on our backs. We had a great time and enjoyed the family experience. We had bicycled across the United States in 1978, but we are now considering doing it again with the children."

"We have raised our baby the 'hard way'—no baby swings, no pacifiers, and seldom am I out of her sight. Everyone tells me how carefree and easy those babyswings are and say that I am making life harder without one. I don't tell them it frightens me to see their baby with a trancelike stare on its face—back and forth, back and forth for an hour! Yikes.

164

Monica has ridden in my back pack as I picked vegetables, canned and froze them. She sits in the flour and squeals at her 'white cloud' as I make bread. I still laugh when I think of her at nine months on my hip as I mashed strawberries in a large bowl. She tried and tried and stretched and tried some more to put her 'piggy toes' in my strawberries!

My husband and I both enjoy the simple things of life. I am happy to afford the luxury of staying home to raise our family. My husband's income is nothing extravagant, but then popcorn, pork and beans, and garden vegetables are good enough for the three of us."

"When I was Director of Pregnancy Aid of Washington State and WIC program for several counties, I realized how difficult it was for many of the women who were working with me to leave their children in daycare. By then all of my children were in school. I established the policy at all Pregnancy Aid offices for both paid and volunteer staff that children could accompany mothers to work. The only stipulation was that the work get done and that the mother make certain the child did not interfere with the work of others.

When our sixth child was born, I took him to work with me from the time he was three weeks old. There were a few raised eyebrows when it was necessary for me to attend meetings at the State Health Department and when I sat breastfeeding, but the program was efficiently and effectively run, and people adapted very quickly. It makes much more sense to me to see those who are involved in the 'work force' adapt to the needs of children than vice versa.

When our seventh child was born, we flew out with the baby for a job interview. We were asked what we would do with our younger children if we were to assume the position. We explained very clearly and carefully that they would, of course, go to work with us. It made no sense to us to be directing programs devoted to the enrichment of marriage and family and to put our children in daycare.

Shortly after taking the job, we found that some people had either not heard or not assumed that we were serious in bringing our children to work, and there was a bit of a question as to whether this would be allowed to continue. We again made it very clear that our children would come to work with us if we were going to work there.

That was two years ago. Our two boys still play (usually quietly) in the corner of our office. There are still some raised eyebrows.

After all, a two-year-old and a four-year-old carrying their lunch pails to work down the corridors of a university is not yet considered usual practice.

I do believe, however, that most parents could take their children to work with them. I have talked with a number of people in the last few years who have seen this practice increasing. One woman has said that in her doctor's office, the nurse brings her infant child to work. Others have mentioned other offices where this is becoming the practice. I realize this is not standard, but I do feel that at every opportunity it should be promoted and that it could become eventually the norm rather than the exception."

"When Molly was eleven months old I received a call from my mother asking me if I would like to accompany her, my father, brother, and sister on a pilgrimage to Mexico City to the Shrine of Our Lady of Guadalupe. There was one stipulation: I would have to wean Molly. My mother did not feel it would work out as far as safety, hotel, traveling, etc. were concerned if I were to bring her along. I gave it a lot of thought and decided that if I could not take Molly along, I would not go. Our nursing relationship meant too much to me. When my mother saw how determined I was and how much it meant to me, she agreed that I could bring the baby along.

We flew to Mexico City while Molly nursed and slept the whole time. Molly and I shared a room with my sister at the hotel. I never had to worry about what she ate or what she drank. She never got sick as many tourists do from the food and water.

I carried her in a cloth baby carrier as we toured the city. She was as good as gold; the people there stopped me on the streets to look at her. If I got tired there were plenty of willing family members to help out. We visited the Shrine, the Pyramids, and several sites throughout the city. We had such a good time."

"When Sarah was only one month old, my husband and I were asked to give talks at the pre-marriage weekends that are held in our town. Since the schedule involved two fairly long days away from home, I could see no possible way of doing the weekends and still being the kind of mother I wished to be.

My husband and I felt that we were 'called' to share our marriage with engaged couples, so after a lot of praying, we found a solution. We hired a babysitter and took Sarah with us. Our babysitter took care of Sarah while we were actually giving talks, and then I was able to nurse her and hold her during breaks and other talks.

An additional benefit that I hadn't realized earlier was that the engaged couples were able to see another important aspect of marriage. No words were needed to tell them that we believed our child was God's most precious gift to us in our marriage. And, of course, we enjoyed showing her off a bit, as any typical parents do!"

"Our small community held a turkey dinner one evening. My husband was working so I took our three-year-old and the baby. When we were being seated, the baby decided he was hungry. The room was packed and we were seated in the middle of a table of middle-aged and elderly people, most of whom I did not know. I knew he would either eat or cry, so I nursed him. Well, one woman filled my three-year-old's plate; another filled mine and even buttered my roll! The only comment was, 'It's so nice to see mothers nursing again.' We all had a wonderful meal and visit.

When our first child was two and a half, we flew to California to visit an aunt who never had children. Her home had white carpeting in one room, and beautiful breakable things through the house. During the visit we ate in restaurants unaccustomed to small children and visited homes of friends with grown children. Although I was somewhat apprehensive about how the visit would go, I knew I'd rather stay home than leave our child. Well, the trip was a success. Sara loved everything, was well behaved, and we received many compliments on her behavior. We let her know what to expect and how to act in each situation, and she really did well.

Our priest and members of our church comment on how well she acts in church. I believe this is partly because I've always taken her to church, and church is one place I expect her to be very, very quiet. If I left her at home or in a nursery until she was two or three or four, then brought her into church, it would be a difficult adjustment.

Looking back, I have never regretted taking my children anywhere. The only regrets and worry I felt were when I left my children and went out alone. I taught school the first year of parenting. Everyone told me over and over that I had the 'ideal' situation. I worked short hours, and went to Grandma's to nurse the baby at noon, and I got a break away from my baby. But for me, it was a terrible year. I never felt I was having a break. My heart was not in my work, but at home. Now that I'm home full-time, I wouldn't trade my position with anyone.

Now I take my children with me everywhere and I enjoy it. I have a friend who cannot shop with her two children because they won't behave. Instead of taking them along to show them how to act, she always leaves them at home. They'll never learn how to shop sitting at home, but only through experiencing it. As I look back over my experiences, I can't help but think of the advice I'd like to give other parents: Please take your children with you. They need to experience different situations, not a babysitter."

16

The Ecology of Natural Mothering

Our attention is often drawn toward the science of ecology and its importance in developing a better world for tomorrow. Man is learning that there is a balance in nature and that when he interferes with this balance, there can be some serious side effects. The environmentalists express their concerns about some issues that affect each one of us. These issues are 1) quality of life, 2) pollution, and 3) population. The environmentalists hold varying opinions on each issue, yet very few have probably considered how breastfeeding could be an "ecological" approach that has wide implications. In all three of these areas our environment could be improved by heeding that most basic form of ecology between mother and baby—breastfeeding. Ecological breastfeeding has many advantages, not only for mother and baby, but also for the wider environment in which they live.

Here it is assumed that ecological breastfeeding means that type of natural mothering described in this book. It excludes that type of breastfeeding commonly observed in our culture which is associated with bottles, pacifiers, mother substitutes, strict schedules, abrupt weaning, and so forth. Secondly, the mother- baby ecology is not limited to breastfeeding, although breastfeeding will be our main concern here. It is obvious that this mother-baby ecology begins at conception, and that it can be disturbed prior to or at the time of birth by man's tamperings.

One of the examples of ecology most familiar to naturalists is relationship between the rhinoceros and the tick bird. The rhino's ticks provide food for the tick bird, and the bird does the rhino a double favor—removing the ticks that bother the rhino and sounding an alarm whenever something approaches. This points up one of the basic facts of ecology: both partners in a natural relationship benefit from it. In the breastfeeding ecology it's not the baby alone who benefits; the mother has her share of blessings also.

QUALITY OF LIFE FOR THE CHILD

No matter what formula and baby food ads would like us to believe, research still shows us that babies thrive best on mother's milk.[1] What happens when man adopts the "scientific" methods of infant feeding? Dr. Otto Schaefer studied the effects of urbanization upon the Eskimos and found that the bottle-fed children had a higher incidence of gastrointestinal diseases, respiratory and middle-ear diseases, and anemia compared to the traditionally breastfed youngsters. He feels strongly that bottle-feeding is related to a very common health problem among children—chronic ear infection. In addition, he states, "Changing infant nutrition practices and the extraordinary perversion of the female breast from a nutritional organ to a sex symbol, which is so typical in Western civilization, has affected the individual's health far beyond infancy, as the markedly higher incidence of allergic and auto-immune diseases in bottle-fed than in breastfed children suggests."[2]

In many of the poorer areas of the world, bottle-feeding has already been introduced, and the protection afforded the baby through breastfeeding has been eliminated. It is known that in these poorer areas where sanitation and food are lacking, the breastfed baby has a lower death rate than the bottle-fed baby. Since the 1960s, experts have been concerned about the value of breastfeeding in these countries for reasons of nutrition, health, and cost.[3]

How does infant technology affect the child emotionally? We now know that a child can suffer according to the degree of maternal deprivation he has experienced during the first few years of life. He may receive the best of physical care with respect to his body, but if he lacks a mother or mother-substitute he does not have the best start in life. An infant thrives on love, security, and intimacy from his mother. By being held, cuddled, and kept in frequent touch with his mother, the child has a richer start than the child who is left with many baby-sitters or allowed to spend hours in an area without the close presence of mother. Maria Montessori stresses the need for mother-baby oneness:

But let us think, for a moment, of the many peoples of the world who live at different cultural levels from our own. In the matter of child rearing, almost all of these seem to be more enlightened than ourselves—with all our Western ultramodern ideals. Nowhere else, in fact, do we find children treated in a fashion so opposed to their natural needs. In almost all countries, the baby accompanies his mother wherever she goes. Mother and baby are inseparable.[4]

An American mother wrote me to explain how she became impressed with a form of mothering she had not witnessed in her own country:

As a college student I majored in intercultural studies and realized many of our child-rearing practices did not seem as successful for either mother or child as those in many non-Western countries...at least in their traditional cultures. I traveled in Africa one summer, and, even though a baby of my own was the farthest thing from my mind, I couldn't help but notice how happy and content all the babies and small children seemed, though I'm certain the general nutrition of their families was usually inadequate. The babies were almost always carried on their mother's backs and children and mothers were together. These facts stayed with me and influenced my attitudes toward our family.

In societies where mother and baby are separate, the rationalization that crying is "good" for a baby seems to develop. Dr. Lee Salk and Rita Kramer discuss this aspect of child raising in their book, *How to Raise a Human Being.*

There's no harm in a child crying: the harm is done only if his cries aren't answered. Babies who are left to cry for long periods of time and are overwhelmed by frustration develop neurotic behavior, in extreme cases even become psychotic. If you ignore a baby's signal for help, you don't teach him independence. How can a helpless infant be independent? What you teach him is that no other human being will take care of his needs.[5]

There are many sayings telling the mother that if her baby receives hate, he will learn to hate. Or if her baby receives love, he will learn to love. This was the basic message of Selma Fraiberg in her *Redbook* article, "How a Baby Learns to Love."[6] She also explains beautifully why the older baby resents a stranger or the separation from mother. Unfortunately, in our society many babies are not learning how to love. They are constantly yelled at, spanked, and shoved around at the will of their parents. And because these children received such treatment, it is likely that they, in turn, will treat their "loved" ones, their spouse and children, in a similar manner. The cases of child abuse are on the uprise, and the evidence shows that the overwhelming majority of these battered children were "wanted" children.

Am I hinting that breastfeeding is going to change all this? No, not automatically, but I seriously think that breastfeeding "the natural way" can bring about many changes. One mother told me that she has spanked her breastfeeding children only once or twice, yet she often spanked her bottle-fed children when they were younger. She felt that she had a greater understanding or sensitivity toward her breastfed children. Another mother said she felt she would be rougher with her child if she didn't breastfeed. Mothers also notice changes in their children's behavior or their parenting behavior once they decide to try the natural mothering program or its associated philosophy of being in tune to the child's needs. Examples are seen in the following excerpts from two mothers:

Our son is in the "terrible two" stage at this time and we seem to be always yelling and spanking him. The past two days I have catered to his wants totally, and my husband remarked how affectionate and well-behaved he seemed to be and asked jokingly if he were sick. He is not aware of my reading your book or change in attitude. Things go much smoother now, even though I am doing what others would consider spoiling him.

I wanted to say that from my experience as a daughter and mother, natural mothering is the only way to raise children. My father (a doctor) never let my mother get close to me for fear of having a "momma's" baby, even telling her to give up nursing since I cried more often than every three hours. I feel that idea has hurt our relationship today; I am not able to be open to them and confide in them.

As a mother at 19, I tried to follow the typical advice about formulas and schedules and potty training, and became a very frustrated mother to the point of shaking and spanking my child. After four more babies I gradually changed. I nursed the last one and really learned how to enjoy all of them. As for my parents, they were ready to pack their bags and go home once when I tried to rock and hold our eight-year-old while she was having a temper tantrum. Thanks for listening.

In other cultures where breastfeeding is common, it is noted that the mother does not hit her child violently, and yet she disciplines. A 1972 *National Geographic* described a society in which affection is the permeating force and violence is lacking.[7] The article notes that the women breastfed for several years and that the mothers are firm when disciplining their children but do not spank them.

In the oneness relationship found in breastfeeding, how can the mother strike or be violent with her child? It is as unlikely as a mother who would strike or mishandle her-self. Lucky indeed is the child who is nursed for several years, for his mother will probably have a close relationship with him that will remain even after the breast-feeding days are gone. He will be loved, and his mother will have learned easily how to respect his needs and his person during the years to come.

Breastfeeding provides a wonder-ful opportunity for physical contact between mother and baby. The importance of a mother's loving touch has especially been revealed in some difficult cases where it has apparently resulted in start-ling improvements in the child's behavior.

In one case a baby approached death as his blood sugar level dropped to zero soon after child-birth. With emergency care he survived, but it was believed that brain damage had occurred. The parents, however, were encour-aged by their doctor, who explained that with the best of care the brain, especially of a newborn, could be reprogrammed.

After a two-week stay in the hospital, the baby—who could just lie there, having lost almost all the responses normal to a small baby—was allowed to come home. Even though he sucked poorly from the bottle filled with breast milk, the mother gradually taught him to nurse at the breast. But what is most impressive is the beautiful care this baby was fortunate enough to receive. The mother says:

In additon to the breastfeeding, David always slept with me and was con-stantly carried, either in my arms or in a Happy Baby Carrier on my chest. Every evening, after the other children were in bed, I would take off all his clothes and play with him, caressing every part of his body, particu-larly his head. He also had a leisurely bath each morning, during which there was a great deal of physical contact. Gradually he began to respond and cry and react like a normal baby.[8]

Upon pediatric examination and neurological testing at five months of age, the child, who had been fed on mother's milk only, was found to be completely normal, and there was no evidence of

The Ecology of Natural Mothering 173

permanent brain damage. The specialists could not believe that this was the same child who had been so sick as a newborn.

Does nature have the answer to child care? It may be worth a try. More writers are stressing the importance of the first few years of life—the importance of the mother-baby relationship, the importance of the mother responding to her baby's cries or fussiness and loving him dearly without fear of spoiling him. On the contrary, they stress the fact that many babies or young children did not receive enough cuddling and holding. Some experts are now devising programs so that children who are having behavioral problems in school can learn touching in a positive sense to build up their self-esteem. It is believed that these children lacked touching or stimulation when necessary for normal development.[9] Frances Cress Welsing, a Washington psychiatrist, claims that many children receive "too little lap time."[10] Welsing believes that the lack of lap time during the early years leads youngsters later into premature sex, drugs and alcohol. She feels that little ones suffer when their mothers work or are too busy to take the time to hold them and thus their emotional needs are not satisfied.

More institutions are recognizing the importance of touching in caring for the sick. Some hospitals are adopting policies that encourage parents and grandparents to touch or cuddle their premies or sick babies. Volunteer "cuddler" programs are also being instituted to provide touching and holding for extremely sick babies whose parents are unable to be there. Such a program at the University of New Mexico Hospital in Albuquerque involves volunteers who provide two to three hours of constant loving care for a very sick baby. Ginny Munsick-Bruno, an occupational- therapist who started the program, claims the research has shown that "it's real important for the baby's mental health and physical development that the environment be responsive to the baby's signals."[11] These volunteers provide the responsive environment.

Other institutions are also practicing an individualized treatment of loving care. I was privileged to witness this type of care among the non-ambulatory, profoundly handicapped children at St. Joseph's Infant and Maternity Home in Cincinnati where one of our daughters became a volunteer. When the nun told the histories of these children and how they outlived their predicted life span for their particular illness, you knew where the answer lay. The volunteers were assigned to one child only and upon each visit spent two hours with "his" or "her" child. Most of the two hours was spent holding the young resident in one's lap or offering personal stimulation by loving and touching. During the summer months, the volunteer held his child in the outdoor pool as these children love water. Smiles were commonly observed on the faces of staff and volunteers. I left my visit feeling very happy for these "special" children and was impressed with the love that permeated their "home." I wondered how much better this world would be if children could receive this same type of wonderful care from their own parents, especially during their formative years.

Once again, the natural nurturing plan provides this same constant responsive care when a mother is always with her baby, nursing frequently and responding to his needs and accomplishments with lots of love. Breastfeeding is an excellent way for a little one to receive lots of lap time, cuddling, and touching in a positive, loving environment. The support and loving care of the dad toward his wife and child is also invaluable to the child's emotional development.

QUALITY OF LIFE FOR THE MOTHER

The mother's own health benefits from breastfeeding. The breastfeeding mother reduces her chance of developing breast cancer; the greater the number of children nursed and the longer the nursing period, the more protection is afforded. Breastfeeding is the natural method of releasing the placenta after birth. A nursing mother does not usually experience the "after-childbirth blues." Nor will she experience a similar fate later under the natural weaning program since the hormonal changes occur very gradually. A nursing mother also regains her prenatal shape faster, especially her internal organs, and in a few cases breastfeeding may prevent surgery. One such lucky mother from Australia wrote as follows:

I suffered a third-degree prolapse of the uterus after the birth of our fourth child. The doctor suggested at only three weeks, then again at six weeks, after birth that I arrange immediately for surgery. I declined on the grounds that it would force weaning onto the baby as well as upset the general family balance. When he saw my reason was genuine, he agreed with my course of action and told me to grin and bear it as long as I could. Well, after four weeks the symptoms ceased to be hurtful and I gradually forgot its presence. At ten months I had occasion to have another doctor do an examination of the cervix. Out of curiosity I asked for his comment on the prolapse; it turned out to be virtually disappeared. He heartily agreed with my suggestion that breastfeeding was the main help in restoring the sagging sinews and muscles to original condition.

It is a well-known fact that nursing often after childbirth is nature's way of contracting the uterus back to its original size. The shots and pills given after delivery for this purpose are normally not necessary for the alert nursing mother.

It is also known that women have a higher iron requirement due to their monthly menses. Television ads frequently encourage women to take iron pills to maintain health and energy. Again, with good nutrition and natural mothering these pills would largely be unnecessary. Through the prolonged absence of menstruation following childbirth, a woman regains her bodily store of iron which would otherwise be lost through menstrual flow. As usual, if we look to nature we will find an answer, and thus lactation amenorrhea is a health asset to the mother in her child-bearing years.

Another physical aspect that is often forgotten in our busy world is the tranquilizing effect that nursing has on a woman. It provides brief rests during the day, and this form of relaxation can be a "plus factor" for the mother who tends to be tense and nervous. In addition, her body is producing prolactin, a "mothering" hormone that bottle-feeding mothers don't have. Thus, the nursing mother is not only **thinking** of being a good mother, but her body is producing the mood and she is **feeling** it as well.

Can breastfeeding be emotionally satisfying and provide fulfillment to the mother within the home?

Today, women's liberation is a popular discussion topic, and one of the big pushes within the movement is to encourage women to seek fulfillment outside the home. In fact, many articles claim motherhood is a myth or that a woman "should" or "must" seek fulfillment outside the home if she is to be happy, if she is to maintain a happy marriage, and so on. The modern woman who desires a family is encouraged to have all three goals: marriage, career, and children. Taking time-out from the business or professional world to raise children is rarely encouraged as the right path for women to follow.

It appears to me that **mother's** "liberation" occurred via the bottle. Mothers looked to the bottle as a way of liberation; it was to free the mother to go more places and do more things. And so the bottle became popular. The baby also became less and less happy, and soon toys and equipment were resorted to in an effort to entertain the baby while mother was being entertained or seeking fulfillment elsewhere. Others rationalized this mother- baby separateness by the "crying-it-out" theory. What has developed is a society in which parents go out of their homes, completely disregarding the fact that they are parents. Go to any women's or mothers' clubs or organizations (except for groups that promote the natural, such as childbirth or breastfeeding) and you will hardly find one mother with her baby. Yet, if mothers read what is being written today, they should have their babies with them regardless of the method of feeding chosen. I might add that the first couple we knew who took their baby with them to all social gatherings were bottle-feeding parents; their baby was an especially good baby. This was in 1970 and I was deeply impressed with this couple's commitment to parenting.

Usually mothering associated with bottle-feeding has liberated women too much from the satisfaction they should naturally derive from being a woman and mother. The bottle has taken away many of her womanly privileges; it has taken away some of the pleasures of mothering. In addition, it has increased the chances of sickness for her baby, taken away the natural infertility designed for her by nature, caused her more work, and cost her more money. Ask any mother who has bottle-fed and breastfed what the difference is between the two methods. I have yet to hear anyone with both experiences rave about the bottle method. The more naturally a mother cares for her baby, the more she will derive enjoyment from it.

What truly liberates a woman is natural or ecological breastfeeding. What she needs to be liberated from today is the cultural pressure to use bottles, pacifiers, and baby foods and to leave her baby at home. She needs to be liberated from the hospital that "owns" the baby, from the doctor who says, "You do as I say or else," from the relatives who fear she will starve the baby, and from a society that promotes working mothers and child-care centers, thus pressuring mothers to work even when it is not a financial necessity. She needs to be liberated from any pressure that contradicts her natural mothering role. What she truly needs is support from relatives, friends, working peers, doctors and church groups.

Liberation via the bottle truly ties a mother down to gadgets and to the expectations of others that she should use whatever technology has made available. The liberation that we should be striving for today is natural mothering, that type of baby care which offers the woman advantages, including the personal satisfaction that a woman can experience only through breastfeeding and the total giving of herself to her baby. It's the type of mothering a woman doesn't want to delegate to another person. It's the type of mothering that gives her a deep feeling of pride in her motherly accomplishments and that may still permeate her attitudes even after her breastfeeding days are over.

Take, for example, the problem of the tired child having difficulty going to sleep. I have known mothers who used strict words, physical threats, candy bars, and even aspirins to get their child to sleep. Yet the natural approach is so much easier--the giving of self in time by lying with the child, rubbing his back, rocking him, singing a soft, slow song, and so on. This approach gives the mother a sense of well-being since she knows that her personal efforts and care helped soothe her child into a deep sleep. The mother who breastfeeds is, I would think, more inclined to give of herself later as she did in the earlier days.

Since we're speaking of quality of life, I would like also to emphasize that much of the richness and happiness in life comes from giving. Too many women today are too concerned about their careers or outside accomplishments at the expense of their husbands, families, the unborn, and the young baby or child. Personal fulfillment is the goal. With breastfeeding, however, I feel that a woman learns that true fulfillment comes in the giving and not the taking. Being human, we know that we have to work at developing certain virtues; no one is naturally good or loving. We think of ourselves or we lose patience with others. It is a continual job to put ourselves at the service of others and to develop better traits. With breastfeeding it might be said that the maturity and character development of the mother can be formed in a very gradual and easy manner. Breastfeeding becomes a learning process whereby the mother learns to think of others—in this sense her children—and to develop certain virtues that will aid her during her entire mothering career.

POLLUTION

The environmentalists should take an interest in advocating breastfeeding, since it does not contribute to the pollution of our air or water, nor does it detract from the environment. Bottle-feeding involves the throwing away of certain items such as bottles, bottle liners, nipples, pacifiers, baby jars, cereal boxes, sterilizers, formula cans, bottle brushes, and so forth. In addition, bottle-feeding entails the use of fuel and water in the preparing, heating, or sterilizing of the milk or food and the cleansing of the equipment to be used.

In our affluent society, we commonly observe the discarding of good clothes. Clothes that could be mended with a good patch or new zipper are simply thrown in the trash. With bottle-feeding, a considerable number of good baby clothes and plastic bibs are likely to be discarded during the early months after childbirth. Juices stain baby clothes so that they are soon unpresentable and are therefore discarded although still not worn. With a breastfed baby, no clothes are stained. You can dress your baby up for a special occasion without worrying about food stains ruining the outfit. Another mother claimed it's ecologically best for mother's clothes, too; she noted that her bottle babies ruined her good clothes when they spit up milk, whereas her breast babies' milk wiped off easily without leaving an odor. She enjoyed not having to wash or dry clean her clothes as frequently as in the past.

With natural breastfeeding there would also be some decrease in the usage of sanitary napkins since mothers would be averaging over a year without menstruating after childbirth. Likewise, there would be a decrease in sales of bottle-related items, which would lower their production and thus decrease the amount of pollution connected with such production. There is no doubt that natural breastfeeding could have a favorable impact toward a better tomorrow from an environmental standpoint.

Other couples carry their interest in ecological breastfeeding to the wider area of natural family planning. One nursing mother who identified herself as not being affiliated with any religious group wrote as follows:

The reason that I am greatly enthused about natural family planning and will use it to the exclusion of any artificial method of contraception, is not because of religious or moral reasons, but because of health reasons. Artificial contraception is yet another way of pollution. It pollutes the body just as our city water and air, the many additives in our foods and bottle-feeding do. You are aware of the fact that with the ecology movement more and more people are becoming interested in antipolluting ways of living in every form possible. Birth control will be no exception. Let's hope that eventually natural family planning will be used by all those interested in keeping themselves, and the future generations, as pure as possible.

POPULATION

No one needs this book to acquaint herself with the population situation in various places throughout the world. However, more attention needs to be given to the role that ecological breastfeeding can play in the birthrate. The decline in breastfeeding should be seen as an important factor in the increased birthrates among some of the developing peoples of the world, and the presence of long-term ecological breastfeeding must be recognized as a key factor in the low birthrates of some primitive peoples.

A neighbor, upon watching a TV special on the Tasadays in the Philippines, was anxious to come over and tell me how long they breastfed their children and how the research people were amazed at their low birthrate. She, of course, immediately suspected that breastfeeding played a big factor in the low birthrate because the children are nursed into their early childhood. These were the same people referred to earlier in this chapter as having an absence of violence in their lives.

A Canadian research doctor has expressed concern about the relationship between breastfeeding and the population increase in some countries. Dr. Otto Schaefer claims that prolonged lactation of about three years among the Eskimos kept the family size small, and that the availability of bottles and milk condensates to the Eskimos via trading posts changed the fertility patterns immensely.

As something of a diversion while I was in Baffin Island in the mid-1950's, I made calculations that indicated that the intervals between siblings shrank in direct relation to the mileage of the family from the trading posts. The shorter the distance, the more frequently they had children. The effect of rapid development of communications and the consequent movements of former camp Eskimos into large settlements is reflected in the more than 50 percent jump in the Eskimo birthrate in the Northwest Territories alone, and the increase from less than 40 births per 1000 in the mid-1950's to 64 per 1000 ten years later. In fact, it is seldom realized that in the last 20 years the Eskimos' population explosion has been as great as or greater than that which has occurred in any developing nation in the world. This is due less to the reduction in infant mortality than to the jump in birthrate. And it is far more intense for the urbanized Eskimo than for those who still live in the scattered hunting camps. There is a clear relationship between the increasing use of bottle feeding and the shortening of lactation. This important point is usually overlooked in searches for explanations of the population explosion seen in developing countries.[12]

In 1960 and 1971 Dr. J. A. Hildes and Dr. Schaefer conducted studies on the Igloolik Eskimos. One outstanding observation dealt with the difference in the fertility rates among the older women as opposed to the younger women due to the change in mothering practices. Women aged thirty to fifty years who had traditionally breastfed for two to three years conceived twenty to thirty months after childbirth, whereas the younger mother under thirty years of age who bottle-fed conceived two to four months after childbirth. These doctors noted that other researchers attribute the population explosion in other countries to a reduced mortality rate. However, the Iglooliks have had a population increase in spite of their high infant death rate. The doctors found that it is the rapid urbanization of these Eskimos during the past twenty years that is responsible for the increase in births, urbanization that brought rapid communication and the rapid introduction of the baby bottle to these people. Thus they lost the natural population control that prolonged breastfeeding had previously given them.[13]

Dr. R. V. Short from Scotland has presented papers on the lactation phase of reproduction and has claimed that "throughout the world as a whole, more births are prevented by lactation than all other forms of contraception put together."[14] Dr. Peter Howie from the United Kingdom claims that for many areas "breastfeeding offered more protection than all methods of contraception combined." In his talk at the Fourth National and International Symposium on Natural Family Planning in November of 1985, Dr. Howie gave a fascinating research statistic. Even when breastfeeding offered only four to eight months infertility, it has been demonstrated that breastfeeding provided 31-1/2 million couple-years of protection. This means 31.5 million couples did not conceive in a single year due to breastfeeding. This is greater "protection" than all the unnatural forms of birth control (condoms, IUD, pills, etc.) put together which was estimated at 24 million couple-years of fertility protection. Howie is convinced that the population increased drastically during the last 1000 years because of artificial baby milk and baby food.[15]

Natural mothering isn't going to cure all of the problems of the world, but it does have some far-reaching effects. At the family level, it contributes to the physical and emotional health of both mother and baby. At the larger community level, it results in less pollution in a number of ways; and at the level of both the individual family and the world, it provides a natural form of birth regulation. With all this going for natural mothering, it would seem more than appropriate that it be encouraged at every level.

Summary of Natural Mothering, Breastfeeding and Child Spacing Program

BASIC PRINCIPLES

1. Frequency of nursing is the primary factor in producing natural lactation amenorrhea and infertility.

2. Natural mothering almost always provides this frequent nursing. By natural mothering, we mean that type of baby care which follows the natural ecology of the mother-baby relationship. It avoids the use of artifacts and follows the baby-initiated patterns. It is characterized by the items in phases I and II below.

PHASE I OF NATURAL MOTHERING (MOTHER ONLY)

This phase almost invariably produces infertility as long as the program is complete. What's in the program?

- Use of the breast for total nourishment and pacification
- Frequent nursing
- Sleeping with baby (night feedings)
- Absence of schedules
- Absence of bottles or pacifiers or cups
- Absence of any practice that restricts nursing or separates mother and baby
- Total breastfeeding in the early months

PHASE II OF NATURAL MOTHERING (MOTHER PLUS OTHER SOURCES)

- Begins when baby starts taking solids from the regular table.
- Liquids are begun later—again when baby begins to show an interest in the cup.
- Use of the breast for pacification, frequent nursing, sleeping with baby, and night feedings.
- The absence of bottles, pacifiers or other practices which restrict the baby's nursing.
- Continues over a period of a year or two or more until baby gradually loses interest in nursing.
- Includes what may be a long period when the baby will be nursing much more for emotional than nutritional nourishment.
- Phase II is a very gradual program in which the **amount** of nursing is 1) not decreased at all at first, and 2) lessened only gradually at baby's pace.
- Phase II begins as soon as baby receives **any** food or liquid other than mother's milk.
- Frequently Phase II will be longer than Phase I with regard to natural infertility **if** the natural mothering program is followed with continued frequent and unrestricted nursing.

CHANCE OF PREGNANCY

For the nursing mother there is about a six percent chance of pregnancy occurring prior to the first menses assuming no fertility awareness and unrestricted intercourse. This risk can be reduced to close to one percent through the techniques of systematic natural family planning—observing the signs of approaching fertility and abstaining accordingly.

NATURAL SPACING BY BREASTFEEDING ALONE

For those couples who desire eighteen to thirty months between the births of their children, "natural mothering" should be sufficient.

FOR MORE EXTENDED SPACING

See Chapter 17, "Natural Family Planning."

References

1. Derrick B. Jelliffe and E. F. Patrice Jelliffe, editors, "The Uniqueness of Human Milk," *The American Journal of Clinical Nutrition,* 24(August 1971):968-1024. This is a collection of eight papers constituting a symposium. Reprints of the entire collection are available and provide a starting point for anyone doing serious research on breastfeeding. Individual copies may be obtained from the CCL office; for bulk copies, contact the offices of the *AJCN.*

2. Otto Schaefer, "When the Eskimo Comes to Town," *Nutrition Today*, November-December 1971, p. 16.

3. Alan Berg, "The Economics of Breastfeeding," *Saturday Review*, May 1973, pp. 29-32. The article provides an excellent short treatment of the dollar and human costs of bottle-feeding on a world-wide basis. It is adapted from *The Nutrition Factor*, The Brookings Institution, 1973.

4. Maria Montessori, *The Absorbent Mind*, (New York: Dell, 1967), p. 104.

5. Lee Salk and Rita Kramer, *How to Raise a Human Being* (New York: Random House, 1969) p. 65.

6. Selma Fraiberg, "How a Baby Learns to Love," *Redbook*, May 1971.

7. Kenneth MacLeish and John Launois, "The Stone Age Men of the Philippines," *National Geographic*, August 1972.

8. Donald Parker, "David's Story," *La Leche League News*, March-April 1971.

9. Sidney B. Simon, "Please Touch! How to Combat Skin Hunger in Our Schools," *Scholastic Teacher*, October 1974, pp. 22-25.

10. William Raspberry, "Preventing Some Social Ills," *The Cincinnati Enquirer*, July 1, 1985.

11. Jim McElroy, "Cuddlers Provide Tender Loving Care," *The Cincinnati Enquirer*, July 11, 1985, p. c-5.

12. Otto Schaefer, *op. cit.,* p.16.

13. J. A. Hildes and O. Schaefer, "Health of Igloolik Eskimos and Changes with Urbanization" (Paper presented at the Circumpolar Health Symposium, Oulu, Finland, June 1971).

14. R. V. Short, "The Evolution of Human Reproduction," *Proc. R. Soc. Lond.* 195(1976)3-24.

15. Peter Howie, "Synopsis of Research on Breastfeeding and Fertility," *Breastfeeding and Natural Family Planning*, ed. Mary Shivanandan (Bethesda, MD: KM Associates, 1986) pp. 7-22.

17

Natural Family Planning

Response to the earlier editions of *Breastfeeding and Natural Child Spacing* included many requests for further information about natural family planning. Many couples see a logical package that includes natural childbirth, natural breastfeeding, and natural family planning. My husband and I go farther and see natural family planning as the only real answer to the technological invasion of human sexuality, love and procreation. Technological man may succeed in his efforts to separate sex and procreation completely. Technology can give freedom from the risk of pregnancy, freedom to have unlimited sexual intercourse, freedom from carrying a child for nine months, and, of course, freedom from that old-fashioned mammarian activity called breastfeeding. However, such "technological freedoms" do not help a person develop as a human being.

Our convictions have been fortified by the realization of how two of the most popular forms of birth control operate. There is no reasonable doubt that the primary mechanism of the IUD (intra-uterine device) is to prevent the newly conceived human life from implanting in its mother's uterus. That is, it acts as a very early abortion agent and so is called an abortifacient.

The birth control pill also has an abortifacient potential. While the combined estrogen-progesterone Pill suppresses ovulation most of the time, it still allows "breakthrough ovulation" to occur. Peel and Potts estimate that breakthrough ovulation occurs in two to ten percent of cycles.[1] A Dutch gynecologist found that with low dosage pills, "in only 20 percent of subjects could no follicular activity be demonstrated, and in 30 percent of subjects follicular growth occurred in all cycles investigated." She also found proof of ovulation in 4.7 percent of all cycles without any increase in recorded pregnancies.[2] ("Follicular growth" refers to the pre-ovulatory development of the ovarian follicle containing an ovum.)

The abortifacient effect of the Pill is caused by the Pill's effect on the inner lining of the uterus. To put it in simple terms, normally the inner lining begins building up after your period stops so that it will provide a rich and plush environment for the implantation of a newly conceived life. However, the Pill throws the normal uterine development out of kilter, resulting in a shriveled up, hostile environment.

The bottom line on the Pill is this: with breakthrough ovulation occurring roughly five percent of the time, the Pill may be acting as an early abortifacient in any given cycle in any given woman. Using a five percent breakthrough ovulation rate and standard probability-of-conception rates for any given cycle (.25 to .50) my husband arrived at this conclusion: there is a high probability that the abortifacient odds will catch up with any individual woman on the Pill within three to five years—some earlier and some later. Another way of looking at it is this: how many women would take a birth control drug that had a high probability of killing **them** within three to five years?[3]

I know this is very hard to hear for many women, and I don't like to say it for that reason. However, the philosophy in back of this book is one of fostering each infant's right to love, care, and the best nutrition. We are only being consistent when we shrink from any method of family planning that would kill a human being even if he is only a few days old and not yet securely settled in his mother's womb.

While we acknowledge that there are many who apparently look for man's technology to give us a better way of doing things than God supplied in the natural ways, we disagree. To assist people who think along similar lines, this book on breastfeeding has been written.

Just as there has been much ignorance about breastfeeding both in general and with special reference to natural child spacing, so is there much ignorance about natural family planning. It is said it is not reliable. That is a half truth. Couples who are ill-informed or who choose to ignore the signs of fertility will have unforeseen pregnancies, but for couples who are well-informed and who live by what they know, natural family planning is highly effective and reliable. Furthermore, our correspondence indicates that many couples have found their marriage enriched when they switched from contraception to natural family planning.

Of particular importance for the nursing mother in this regard is the observation of cervical mucus. As we noted in an earlier chapter, the available evidence indicates that about 94 percent of nursing mothers will experience menstruation before achieving pregnancy again. To find out if she is in that small group for whom fertility comes before her first menses, the nursing mother can examine herself for the cervical mucus which is part of nature's preparation for pregnancy since it aids sperm life and migration. In *The Art of Natural Family Planning*[4], my husband and I describe how this mucus changes in consistency and what this means in terms of fertility. Suffice it to say that the well-informed mother can detect the onset of fertility even before her first postpartum menstruation. Furthermore, she can nurse as long as she and the baby desire and still practice natural family planning successfully.

SOME BASIC PHYSIOLOGY

The normal fertility cycle is much better understood than the relationship between nursing and its effect upon fertility. What follows is a simplified version of what happens, and it's not intended to be an instruction in how to practice natural family planning; however, it will give you a basic understanding of your normal fertility cycle and how that knowledge is used in modern NFP.

A few days after your period stops, but sometimes sooner, your brain tells your pituitary gland, a small organ at the base of your brain, to send out a signal that says, "Let's ovulate." That pituitary hormone is called FSH, follicle stimulating hormone, and it stimulates a follicle in one of your ovaries to begin to develop. (The ovary is your "egg basket," and each egg is contained in an individual follicle.) As the follicle develops, it secretes estrogen, a basic female hormone that has several important effects. The first of these you can't see: it causes the inner lining of the uterus to develop. It also has two more effects that you can see or experience. First of all, estrogen causes some cells in the cervix to secrete a mucus discharge which is very necessary for normal fertility. (The cervix is the lower end of the uterus that protrudes slightly into the vagina.) This mucus starts out as a rather tacky or sticky substance and then typically becomes like raw egg white. Its function is to aid sperm life and migration; your mucus discharge is a very positive sign that you are fertile, i.e., that relations at this time could result in pregnancy.

Estrogen also causes physical changes in the cervix itself. It tends to rise slightly, the mouth of cervix (the cervical os) opens just a bit, and the tip becomes softer.

You can notice the mucus both at the outer lips of the vagina and at the cervical os; the changes in the cervix are observed by an internal exam. Some women find they get very adequate information from the external observation of the cervical mucus at the outer lips of the vagina; others find the internal observation more helpful.

After about a week of FSH and estrogen activity, ovulation occurs: an egg is released from an ovary and is picked by a fallopian tube to start its journey toward the uterus. If you have relations at the fertile time, sperm and egg can meet in the tube; their union is called conception or fertilization, and the result is a new human being. If conception occurs, about a week later your newly conceived baby implants in your uterus.

After ovulation, the follicle that released the egg gets a new look and a new name: it becomes yellowish and is called the **corpus luteum**, Latin for yellow body. The corpus luteum secretes the second basic female hormone, progesterone, and this hormone has several effects on the fertility cycle. First of all, it maintains the inner lining of the uterus and gives it a rich blood supply in preparation for possible implantation. Secondly, it causes your temperature to rise slightly but noticeably; thirdly, in conjunction with decreased levels of estrogen, it causes the mucus discharge to stop and the cervix changes to reverse—it becomes lower and firmer and the opening closes.

The bottom line is this: there are three commonly recognized signs of fertility and infertility—mucus, temperature and cervix. You can learn to observe these; you can use two or three of them together in a crosschecking way—the Sympto-Thermal Method, or you can use single-sign systems such as mucus-only or temperature-only. You can use this information both to achieve and to avoid pregnancy; you can use it in normal or irregular cycles, and you can also use it to monitor the return of fertility while breast-feeding.

THE TYPICAL CYCLE

In a typical cycle, this is what you would experience. After a menstrual period of about five days, you would probably have two or three "dry days"—days without any mucus. Then you would notice the beginning of the mucus discharge—usually rather sticky or tacky at first—and the opening of the cervix, if you're making that observation. Those are positive signs that the fertile time has started. Next you would notice the mucus becoming like raw egg white and/or producing distinct feelings of wetness on the outer lips, and this would last for a few days. Finally, you would notice the mucus disappearing and that your waking temperature was rising. Typically, on the third day of well elevated temperatures and drying up of the mucus, you would be into the time of postovulation infertility, and you couldn't become pregnant even if that was your greatest desire.

And, speaking of the desire to become pregnant, the techniques of NFP are being used by more and more couples in the conscious effort to achieve pregnancy. Part of it is knowing the best possible timing; and part of it is learning things you can do about your eating, exercise, and lifestyle to enhance your fertility. If you achieve pregnancy, your temperature will remain elevated. The upward shift in temperature after ovulation remains the single best way to estimate gestational age and the date of childbirth; after three weeks of elevated temperatures you have a 99% certainty that you are carrying another gift of the Lord.

If pregnancy was not achieved in that cycle, the corpus luteum stops secreting progesterone after 12-14 days; the lining of the uterus can no longer be sustained, and it is sloughed off in the process of menstruation.

EFFECTIVENESS OF NATURAL FAMILY PLANNING

How effective is NFP as a method to avoid pregnancy and which form of NFP is best for that purpose? The U. S. Federal Government was asking that question in the seventies and ran a study from 1976 to 1978 at a Jewish hospital in Los Angeles to compare the Sympto-Thermal Method (STM) with a mucus-only method frequently called the Billings Ovulation Method (BOM).[5] Couples were randomly assigned to either side of the study; i.e., they couldn't pick which side they wanted to be in. The study revealed that the couples in the Sympto-Thermal side did better: of those who followed the STM rules for avoiding pregnancy, zero became pregnant; in the mucus-only group, there was a 5.7 percent unplanned pregnancy rate. This and other studies provide the basis for the statement that the Sympto-Thermal Method has a method effectiveness of 99 percent.

Of course, there were also couples who, for one reason or another, didn't follow the rules. In that group, the STM people also did better: they had an unplanned pregnancy rate of 15.2 percent, while the BOM group had an unplanned pregnancy rate of 37.3

percent. Both methods have shown much better results in other studies; I am quoting the Los Angeles study because it is the only American **comparative** study on record, and that American comparison is part of the reason why the Couple to Couple League teaches the Sympto-Thermal Method. However, it is taught in such a way that any couple who would prefer to use a single-sign system can do so.

It's not just that human fertility is now so well understood; what is really important is that the academic knowledge has been put to use. Never before in human history has it been so easy for so many couples to learn their own times of fertility and infertility.

In the effort to spread the knowledge about systematic natural family planning as well as ecological breastfeeding, in 1971 my husband and I founded the Couple to Couple League for natural family planning. Professionally trained volunteer teaching couples now teach NFP courses in 48 American states and several European and Latin American countries, but the service network is far from completion. So, for couples who do not live near teachers, we have developed a home study course. Every couple who can read this book in English can teach themselves systematic natural family planning with the *CCL Home Study Course*.

As I mentioned earlier, once you understand your normal fertility pattern and what your normal cervical mucus is like, then you're in a great position to understand the signs of returning fertility while you're breastfeeding. With that understanding you'll almost always be able to detect your return of fertility even if it occurs before you have a first "warning" period.

Can you learn to detect the signs of fertility if you're learning about this for the first time while you're pregnant or breastfeeding? Very definitely, yes. Certainly it's easier to learn during normal cycles, but while you are pregnant or breastfeeding you can learn what to be looking for and know it when you experience it. Thousands before you have already done it.

However, the above general description is not intended to prepare you inadequately to detect and properly evaluate your signs of fertility and infertility. You would be silly to try to practice any form of systematic NFP or to think you are well prepared to detect your return of postpartum fertility based on the brief description above. Learning NFP is something like learning to tie your shoes. It looks simple at first, then it looks complicated as you get into it, and then it becomes simple once you have mastered it. To help couples achieve the mastery they need, we have developed both a teaching program and the home study course. Both the classes and the home study course use *The Art of Natural Family Planning* as a key ingredient.

For further information, see the Mini-catalog in the back of this book.

References

1. John Peel and Malcolm Potts, M.D., *The Textbook of Contraceptive Practice* (New York: Cambridge University Press, 1969) p. 98.

2. Dr. Nine van der Vange, quoted in "We are close to lowest steroid dosage in the Pill," *News and Views* (Excerpts from Second Annual Meeting of the Society for the Advancement of Contraception in Jakarta, Indonesia, November 26-30, 1984) p.4.

3. For further documentation about the abortifacient properties of the IUD and the Pill, see these three items: a) "The Pill and the IUD: Some Facts for an Informed Choice;" b) *Birth Control and Christian Discipleship*, pp. 11-13; c) *Silent Abortions* by Lutherans for Life. All are available from the Couple to Couple League.

4. John F. and Sheila K. Kippley, *The Art of Natural Family Planning* (Cincinnati: The Couple to Couple League, 1987).

5. Maclyn E. Wade et al, "A Randomized Prospective Study of the Use-Effectiveness of Two Methods of Natural Family Planning," *Am. J. Ob and Gyn* 141:4(Oct. 15, 1981)368-376.

Appendix I

A Postscript to Husbands

by John F. Kippley

If you are a typical husband, you may not share your wife's enthusiasm for reading books and other literature about breastfeeding. Perhaps your wife has given you this chapter and asked you to read it, so I'll make it brief. I'm just going to share a few thoughts that you might find helpful.

First of all, you can be proud of your wife for breastfeeding your baby. She's doing what is best for him—and for her. Give her support because she needs it from you. She needs to know that you are grateful she's doing what is best for your baby.

Secondly, there are some experiences that you will probably miss, or at least have less of, than the fathers of bottle-fed babies. For one thing if your wife has a prepared, natural childbirth and comes right home from the hospital or birthing center, or if she has a home birth, you won't have the experience of visiting her at the hospital each day for several days. Then, because the breastfed baby has health advantages over the bottle-fed baby, your baby will most likely have fewer illnesses, allergies, and so on, than if your wife had not nursed. You are also going to miss the experience of the horrible mess that is made when mothers (or fathers) try to feed babies solids in the early months. I can still distinctly remember one Saturday morning back in my bachelor days when I stopped to pick up a buddy for golf. He invited me in for a cup of coffee while his wife was feeding a very young baby. I swear that seeing that stuff all over everything—hair, face, arms—scared me into a few more years of bachelorhood. It's an experience I haven't missed at all with our breastfed children. From the above, it is also obvious that you are going to miss the expenses associated with baby foods and increased medical problems.

One thing we have had some questions on is the idea of the baby sleeping in bed with his parents. We have been told of husbands who initiated the idea, and we have also heard from wives telling us that they think their husbands would object to having the baby as sort of an intruder in the marriage bed, that the presence of the baby will interfere with marital intimacy. The most simple answer is that it doesn't. "Sleeping with baby" doesn't mean he's with you all the time. He will normally be asleep before you go to bed, and you can put him in another bed for a while. I'm sure that any couple with a little ingenuity can have their marital intimacy and their "sleeping with baby," too.

Keep in mind that it is your baby's **regular** suckling that brings about breastfeeding's side effect of extended natural infertility. If you train the baby to sleep by himself all through the night, your wife may very well be deprived of the sucking stimulus she needs for continued natural infertility and maybe even for her continued ample milk supply. It also helps to keep in mind that those night nursings are saving you the trouble of getting up for middle-of-the-night bottle warmings.

Being a father calls for a little maturity. The baby is your child, and his needs call for more instant satisfaction than yours. If your wife is preparing dinner and the baby really needs to nurse, don't get upset if dinner is a few minutes late. Don't be afraid to pitch in with the dishes when your baby needs his mother. And finally,

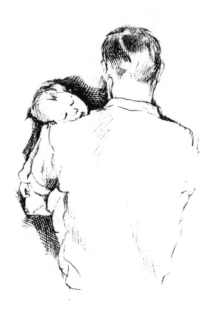

when all that your baby needs is a changing, some holding, some walking, or some rocking, be sure to get in on the act. There is something very satisfying about having your babe fall asleep in your arms.

Support your wife when she allows your child to wean at his own pace. You thought he would never walk—and then he did. You thought he would never talk—and then he did and won't stop. You think he's never going to wean—and he will when he's ready. In other cultures throughout the world it is common for three-year-olds to still nurse occasionally. Your child will be big and older before you know what has happened. Relax and enjoy the nursing years, and you'll be glad you did.

Appendix II

Personal Research

To test the theory that ecological breastfeeding spaces babies for American women just as it does for women in primitive and developing parts of the world, my husband and I have conducted two pieces of research.

The results of the first study were compiled and first presented at the La Leche League International Convention in 1971 and were later published in a nursing journal in 1972[1]. In that study, readers of the first mimeographed edition of this book returned a survey about their breastfeeding experiences. After discarding a few surveys because of insufficient data, we reported the results from 112 nursing experiences of 72 mothers, and most of those experiences had occurred before reading this book.

In both studies we used the first postpartum menstruation as an indication of the return of fertility. We realize that this is not the best marker of fertility; the temperature graph is far superior. Nevertheless, it provides a fairly accurate indicator and is universally applicable.

What we found in both studies confirmed our basic conviction that ecological breastfeeding provides significantly more postpartum infertility than partial or cultural breastfeeding. The results showed that on the average babies will be spaced about two years apart with ecological breastfeeding, assuming random intercourse and no form of conscious birth control.

THE 1971 STUDY

First, we found the average length of amenorrhea of the entire study group: 10.2 months; this included **both** cultural and ecological nursing experiences. Then we selected **six criteria for eco-**

194

logical breastfeeding. These criteria are directly related to practices that increase or decrease the amount of suckling at the breast and are as follows:

1. No pacifiers used
2. No bottles used
3. No liquids or solids for five months
4. No feeding schedules other than baby's
5. Presence of night feedings
6. Presence of lying-down nursing for naps and night feedings.

Duration of amenorrhea

Our analysis showed that 29 of the entire 112 nursing experiences fulfilled all these requirements. These 29 mothers nursed 22.8 months on the average; this was 40 percent longer than the 16.3 months of nursing for the entire sample.

Of great significance, the ecologically breastfeeding group **averaged 14.6 months of breastfeeding amenorrhea**, and this was 43 percent longer than the average of 10.2 months of amenorrhea experienced in the 112 nursing experiences, i.e., the sample as a whole.

Actually, the contrast between those doing ecological breastfeeding and those doing some form of cultural breastfeeding was greater than illustrated by these numbers because the figures for the "sample as a whole" include the ecological nursing experiences. This inclusion raised the averages for the sample as a whole, so in our 1986 study we directly compared the ecological breastfeeding experiences with those of cultural breastfeeding as explained below.

Early return of menses

There were only two cases of menses returning prior to seven months postpartum in our sample of twenty-nine cases of natural mothering. One woman who engaged in the natural mothering program still experienced the return of menses at six weeks postpartum. However, she kept basal temperature charts which her obstetrician interpreted as indicating infertile periods up through the eleventh menses. The second mother, whose menses returned at four months postpartum, also used basal temperature charts which indicated a return of ovulation six or seven months postpartum.

In the entire group of 142 returned questionnaires, there were 14 instances of pregnancy occurring prior to the return of menses. (Eighty-nine of the 142 cases indicated reliance on amenorrhea for conception regulation.) Thirteen of these questionnaires provided enough detail for analysis of baby-care-feeding programs. Of these, only two were among the 29 who followed the program of total natural mothering. One mother conceived at twenty-seven months postpartum, but she had deliberately reduced her nursing in order to conceive; the other mother became pregnant at fifteen months postpartum. The other eleven were from the larger sample whose nursing habits were more typical of the American culture. An analysis in Table I indicates significant factors in their nursing or mothering patterns.

There were no conceptions by any mother in the natural mothering group of 29 prior to the twelfth month, and the earliest conception without a "warning" menses was the fifteenth month as stated above.

Table I: Relationship of nursing patterns to conception in eleven cultural nursing experiences; 1971

Month of conception	Comment
2nd	Began liquids on Day 1, used pacifier
5th	Began liquids at 1 month, solids at 4 months, night feedings for only 3 months
6th	Began solids and liquids at 6 months, no night feedings
7th	Began solids at 3 months, liquids at 6 months, night feedings for only 3 months, no lying down nursing, nursed on a schedule
8th	Solids at 2 months, liquids at 7 months, pacifier used
8th	Weaned at 8 months, conceived before next period
9th	Totally breastfed for 1 month, solids at 4 months (other data insufficient)
11th	Solids at 5 months (no other data)
11th	Solids at 4 months, liquids at 6 months, night feedings for 6 months, used pacifier
12th	Solids at 5 months
14th	Solids at 5 months, used bottle and pacifier, night feedings for 10 months

The 1971 study reinforced the conviction already developed from the research of others. The sample of nursing experiences which fulfilled the criteria for ecological breastfeeding showed that the well fed American mother could experience a duration of breastfeeding amenorrhea that would, on the average, space her babies about two years apart.

THE 1986 STUDY

During the next fifteen years, completed breastfeeding surveys continued to trickle in, and by 1986 we had over 1500 of them. Early that year, CCL teaching couple Oscar and Susan Staudt wrote a data analysis computer program, and 286 surveys were entered for analysis. The surveys used were not pre- selected; our summertime data input clerk simply ran out of time when she had 286 surveys entered, and we decided to run the analysis at that point and to publish the results in the CCL newsletter.[2] Using the same six criteria we used in 1971, we found 98 nursing experiences that qualified as ecological breastfeeding.

Total months of breastfeeding

One of the biggest differences between the two surveys was the average duration of breastfeeding for the entire sample. In the 1986 survey, the 286 nursing experiences averaged 20.4 months, 25 percent longer than the 16.3 average duration in the 1971 survey. We speculate that this increase may be due to two factors: 1) an increased social acceptance of more extended nursing and 2) the influence of reading the earlier edition of this book and the "natural mothering" columns in the newsletter of the Couple to Couple League. As mentioned before, most of the nursing experiences in the 1971 survey occurred before the mothers read an earlier edition of this book, but almost all the 1986 surveys were from CCL newsletter readers because the data-entry clerk started with the batch of survey forms that had been printed in the newsletter. This may have influenced some mothers to nurse longer. The sample of 98 ecological breastfeeding experiences averaged 25.7 months of nursing (compared to 22.8 in 1971).

Duration of amenorrhea

The average duration of amenorrhea for the 286 nursing experiences was 11.7 months (compared with 10.2 in 1971).

The sample of 98 ecological breastfeeding experiences averaged 14.5 months of amenorrhea. We think this was the most important finding of this study because it confirmed the primary finding of the 1971 study where we had found an average of 14.6 months of breastfeeding amenorrhea with ecological breastfeeding. We now have two studies 15 years apart yielding almost identical results on this key point, so we can say with even greater confidence than before that American women who follow the pattern of ecological breastfeeding will experience an average of fourteen and a half months of amenorrhea.

Comparison between ecological and cultural breastfeeding

A comparison was made between the ecological breastfeeding group and the cultural breastfeeding experiences. The results are illustrated in Table II. The total adds up to 284 experiences; inexplicably, two computer records failed to be tallied.

Table II: Comparison of duration of amenorrhea

	Ecological Breastfeeding N = 98	Cultural Breastfeeding N = 186
Average Months of Nursing	25.7	17.5
Average Months of Amenorrhea	14.5	10.3

The ecological breastfeeding mothers averaged approximately 40 percent greater duration of amenorrhea than the cultural breastfeeding mothers.

We then tried to discover if there was any single one of the six criteria we used for ecological breastfeeding that by itself showed an even greater duration of amenorrhea, but we found none. However, three of those criteria showed their significance in contributing to the overall effect:

1) baby not having a pacifier
2) having night feedings
3) sleeping with your baby.

The single factor that correlated most closely with the average amenorrhea for ecological breastfeeding was total nursing for the first **six** months. (The criterion for the ecological breastfeeding sample was total nursing for the first **five** months.) In 79 experiences, the baby took no other nourishment for the first six months, and the mothers averaged 14.8 months of amenorrhea.

However, total breastfeeding usually lasts only for five to seven months unless the baby is experiencing allergies, so the total breastfeeding for six months by this sub-sample by itself could not account for the continuation of amenorrhea for an average of another eight months. Rather, the total breastfeeding for six months or a bit more perhaps indicated a combination of the baby's suckling needs and the mother's attitude towards baby-led introduction of other foods, and this pattern may have carried forward for many months.

Since we were unable to find any single factor which could be effective for 12 months and more, we were confirmed in our conviction that it is a combination of all the elements of natural mothering which results in the side effect of a year or more of natural infertility. To repeat, our research confirms that it is the entire package we call "natural mothering" that spaces babies; it is that form of baby care that results in the Creator's original form of natural family planning.

VARIATION AND POSSIBLE CAUSES

Significant variation in the return of menses continues to be recorded even among mothers doing ecological breastfeeding, and that range is illustrated in Table III.

Table III: Variation in amenorrhea with ecological breastfeeding

Range in months of amenorrhea	Number of experiences (N = 98)	Percent
1-6	7	7
7-12	36	37
13-18	32	33
19-24	15	15
25-30	8	8

Average months of amenorrhea: 14.5

In this sample, in 93% of the cases, there were more than six months of amenorrhea; 56% of the experiences had more than one year of amenorrhea with ecological breastfeeding.

Among mothers who did ecological breastfeeding for 18

months and more, we found that 34% had 18 months or more of amenorrhea. That figure is not immediately evident from Table III; it includes eleven who had 18 months of amenorrhea plus the 23 who had between 19 and 30 months.

We do not know what causes this sort of variation. If two mothers are following the same breastfeeding pattern but one has a return of menses at six months and the other at sixteen, we don't know why. Undoubtedly, some is due to differences in the suckling needs and patterns of different babies. There are probably differences in the response of different women to the same amount of suckling stimulus.

It's also possible that some of this difference may be due to the nutrition and body-build of the mother. This is not a new speculation; for some time researchers have debated the relative significance of suckling versus nutrition. We are convinced that research has shown that the frequency of suckling is the prime ingredient in maintaining breastfeeding infertility, but the variation we have seen in our two American samples raises questions about the secondary effects of nutrition, exercise and body-build of the nursing mother. To pursue these questions, a new breastfeeding survey has been formulated. Mothers interested in participating in this survey may write the Couple to Couple League (P. O. Box 111184, Cincinnati, OH 45211) for the survey questions.

References

1. Sheila K. and John F. Kippley, "The Relation between Breastfeeding and Amenorrhea: Report of a Survey," *JOGN Nursing* 1:4, November-December, 1972.

2. Sheila Kippley, "Breastfeeding Survey Results Similar to 1971 Study," *The CCL News* 13:3 (November-December 1986)10 and 13:4 (January-February 1987) 5.

INDEX

Kenny, James, 20
Kern, Coralee, 66
Kimball, Robbins, 108
Klaus, Marshall, 123
Konner, Melvin, 42
Kramer, Rita, 171
!Kung mother, 42
La Leche League Int., 89, 100
Lambo, Thomas, 48-49
Le Shan, Eda, 116
liberation, women's, 177-78
Livingston, Connie, 98

marital intimacies, 19, 56, 130
McKenna, James, 21-22
Mead, Margaret, 50, 119
menstruation and menstrual cycle,
    5-6, 186-87
  spotting, 78
  weaning and return of, 76-80
midwife, 92, 94
milk and milk supply
  adoptive mothers, 2-3
  colostrum, 93, 95, 104
  expression and, 1-2, 43, 47
  leakage, 129
  nutrition, 104-5
  oversupply and nursing
      problems, 27-28
  sucking and, 1-3
  twins, 3
Moloney, James Clark, 34, 53
Montagu, Ashley, 20
Montessori, Maria, 50, 115, 170
Moss, Stephen, 30
mothering, natural, 6-7, 39-40, 45,
    47 *passim*
  inseparability, 39, 48-52,
      55-57, 71
  marsupial, 53-54
  program summarized, 181-83
mothers
  African, 48-49
  Eskimos, 81, 180
  Gainj, 42
  !Kung, 42
  Rwanda, 56

working, 19, 50, 66-67
Murray, Michael, 129

Nader, Ralph, 97
NAPSAC, Int., 92, 100
natural family planning, 11, 142,
    179, 185-90
  home study course, 189-90
newborn, 93, 95, 104
Newton, Niles, 22, 75
night feedings,
  advantages, 18-22
  attitudes towards, 13-16
  breathing patterns, 21-22
  burping, 18
  infertility, 13, 24, 40-41, 135
  marital intimacies, 19, 56
  nursing in bed, 16-18
  sleeping arrangements, 17
  sudden infant death syndrome,
      20-22
Nighttime Parenting (Sears), 20
nipples
  breast, sore, 86, 130
  sucking differences, breast and
      bottle, 29-30
nursing, infant
  at church, 59, 69
  at restaurants, 63-64
  frequency, 28, 39-44, 53, 74
  in bed, 16
  in public, 58-62, 120
  money saved, 111
  obesity, 107, 109
  total, 8-9, 11, 21, 50, 111-12
  unrestricted, 22, 28, 43
  while taking drugs, 88
  while traveling, 65, 111
Nursing Mother, The
    (Richardson), 110
nursing older child
  attitudes, 124
  experiences, 120-21
  illnesses, 116-17
  night feedings, 121
  reasons for, 115-120
  separations, 122-23

uterus, postpartum, 175-76

A Mini-Catalog

The following is a sample of items which are available through the Couple to Couple League catalog.

The Art of Natural Family Planning by John and Sheila Kippley

The CCL manual which explains the Sympto-Thermal Method of NFP. In addition to the basics, it contains sound reasons for the use of natural family planning, an explanation and defense of ecological breastfeeding and full-time mothering, an entire chapter on the return of fertility after childbirth, and seeking-pregnancy tips for those of marginal fertility. Also in Spanish.

Basic Starter Kit

The basic minimum for learning the method: *The Art of Natural Family Planning*, a practical applications workbook, a year's supply of charts and a thermometer—all in one package.

The Home Study Course

This course contains all you need in order to learn natural family planning very well right in the comfort of your own home. It contains everything in the Basic Starter Kit and much more—starting with a second thermometer to have handy if you break the first. What distinguishes it most from the Basic Starter Kit is *The Home Study Guide to Natural Family Planning*, a book written specifically in how-to-do-it language and directed towards the person who cannot attend NFP classes. (*The Art of Natural Family Planning* was originally written as a supplement for classroom and personal instruction.)

The Home Study Guide breaks the learning process into 30 short lessons. Doing a lesson a day, you will learn all the basics in two weeks, and within a month you can learn even the fine points. The course also includes a review of your first three cycle-charts and CCL's bi-monthly membership newsletter for a year.

E-Z Baby Tote

Babies and parents love this baby carrier. Padded shoulder straps, no leg holes, comfortable, no shoulder stress, washable denim. Baby is carried in front and receives some neck support from the carrier.

Breastfeeding Patterns

Designed for the breastfeeding mother. Comfortable, stylish, multi-sized, they allow for discreet nursing. Many can also be used for maternity. Brochures and prices available upon request.

Other Books

The Womanly Art of Breastfeeding by La Leche League

The basic and complete how-to-do-it manual for the breastfeeding mother.

The Five Standards for Safe Childbearing by David Stewart, Ph. D.

Provides research-backed standards in the areas of nutrition, midwifery, natural childbirth, home birth, and breastfeeding.

Nighttime Parenting by William Sears, M.D.

Points out the merits of the family bed and offers advice for problem situations involving sleep—sleeping disorders, night-waking, SIDS, etc.

The Heart Has Its Own Reasons: Mothering Wisdom for the 1980s by Mary Ann Cahill

Supportive of full-time mothering; offers many suggestions on how to manage on one income. Excellent philosophy of how a simple lifestyle makes for improved family living.

Planning Your Own Home Business by Coralee Smith Kern

Provides expert advice in how to set up and run your own home business, market products and services, target new markets, and get the best use of banking, accounting, insurance and other professional services.

Booklets and Brochures

Birth Control and Christian Discipleship

Recalls the pre-1930 universal Christian biblical teaching against unnatural forms of birth control, the Anglican and Protestant departure from that teaching in 1930, the historic, legal and physiological connections between contraception and abortion, and the whole birth control issue in the light of Christian discipleship.

Breastfeeding: Does It Really Space Babies?

Briefly describes the ecological breastfeeding that spaces babies and how to detect the return of fertility.

The Case for Natural Family Planning

Eight reasons modern couples are choosing natural family planning.

The Effectiveness of Natural Family Planning

Reviews scientific studies which demonstrate the high effectiveness of natural family planning; also describes why this information is not widely known in either the health care community or the general public.

The First Three Years of Life

Quotations from educators, physicians, psychiatrists, and child care experts which show the importance of mother-child togetherness during the first three years of life.

The Pill and the IUD: Some Facts for an Informed Choice

Documentation on the abortifacient properties and health hazards of the Pill and the IUD.

Silent Abortions

An excellent booklet documenting the evidence of the abortifacient actions of the Pill and the IUD. Published by the Illinois-Indiana Chapter of Lutherans for Life.

All of the above are available from the Couple to Couple League. For current prices, request the current catalog from CCL, P. O. Box 111184, Cincinnati OH 45211.

208